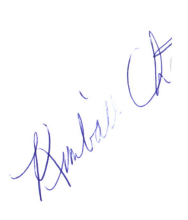

MW01487789

ASTRAGALUS

Ancient Herb
for
Modern Times

Kimball Chatfield O.M.D., L.Ac.

Range of Light Publishing
870 Emerald Bay Road Box 5
South Lake Tahoe, CA 96150

ASTRAGALUS: ANCIENT HERB FOR MODERN TIMES
Copyright 2014 by Kimball Chatfield

Notice
Although extensive time and research has been utilized to determine the accuracy of this text, errors unbeknownst to the author could potentially occur. It is the responsibility of the reader to utilize this information reasonably and cautiously. This is not a substitute for professional diagnosis and treatment. To the fullest extent of the law, neither the publisher or author assume any liability for any injury and/or damage to persons or property arising out of or related to any use of the material contained in this book.

Publisher and author:
Kimball Chatfield

Book Designer:
Kristen Schwartz
KristenSchwartz.com

Cover photos:
Astragalus root © Lcc54613 | Dreamstime.com
Astragalus plant © Kazakovmaksim | Dreamstime.com

For Melinda

TABLE OF CONTENTS

Foreward 1

Introduction.. 4

What is Astragalus?... 7

Astragalus and Diabetes... 16

Astragalus and Immunity 32

Anemia and Leukopenia... 38

Cancer.. 42

Heart Disease 59

The Brain and Nervous System................................ 66

Liver.. 75

Lupus – Systemic Lupus Erythematosus (SLE)......... 78

Aging and Life Extension 80

Healing Injuries... 86

Astragalus and Inflammatory Diseases 91

Using Astragalus 94

References 99

Index... 129

About the Author 135

FOREWARD

I began my formal training in natural health care in the late 1970's in naturopathic medical college. I remember talking with a scientist regarding the idea of utilizing herbal and nutritional therapies to help a person's body become more efficient and healthier in order to prevent and fight disease. He said it sounded somewhat logical but at that time he was concerned that there wasn't enough scientific study into this idea. "Where's the data?," he said. In the 1970's there was a lack of substantial scientific research in many areas of natural healthcare. Now in the 21st century we can say, "The data has arrived." Scientific research technology has evolved enough today so that we can see how cells work at the molecular level. We can even measure the expression or suppression of genes caused by chemicals that we come in contact with every day or as a part of medical intervention. We can see the release of inflammatory and anti-inflammatory chemicals. We can see cells grabbing viruses and presenting them to white blood cells for their destruction. We also now have the data to show how many herbal medicines and nutritional therapies work for a wide variety of diseases.

One of the herbal medicines that has attracted significant research is astragalus. With increased interest also comes myth and confusion. After reading over 1,600 scientific studies on astragalus it strikes me how much misinformation is written and taught regarding astragalus. Even individual research scientists, often looking only at one small area of astragalus research, have failed to grasp the big picture regarding astragalus. One author may find that astragalus increases the creation of blood vessels (called angiogenesis) and another author may say that astragalus reduces angiogenisis. The truth is that astragalus can upregulate angiogenesis to create new vessels to feed the healing of an injury. It can also downregulate and stop the formation of blood vessels to cancerous tumors, starving them.

The big picture that many doctors are missing is that astragalus is an alterative. Alteratives, not to be confused with the word alternative, are medicines that alter the body to move in the direction of health. They increase the efficiency of the body. By being more efficient and "smarter", the body can respond to multiple health problems much better. This concept of a medicine being alterative is often foreign and difficult to appreciate if you are a physician who has been prescribing medicines that move physiology in only one direction.

Astragalus is also an adaptogen. The word adaptogen was coined by Soviet scientist N.V. Lazerev in 1947. In 1958 his student I. Brekhman began giving tonic herbs to soldiers, athletes, and future cosmonauts to help them adapt to the stresses of exercise and space travel. Adaptogens are nutrients that increase our resistance to various stresses such as overwork, injury, contagious illnesses, environmental toxins, etc. with little or no side effects.

Another important consideration is in the actual research itself. Most of Astragalus research is outside the United States. The vast majority of research is from China. This is because medicinal astragalus species grow there and have been used for thousands of years. I have noted significant bias against these studies simply due to the fact that many older Chinese studies can be poorly worded and translated, lacking all of the specific language required by scientists in America. Some American scientists are of the opinion that only American scientific studies are worthy of publication. Because I have worked in this field for over 30 years, I have often seen this prejudice. Many non-scientists might be surprised at the turf battles and egomaniacal arguments that take place in the politics of science. The vast majority of recent Chinese scientific studies on astragalus are well researched and well written.

The general idea that only American scientists can create and produce good research is a canard. American scientists who have this attitude towards foreign researchers should take note that funding for medical research in China is increasing several hundred percent every year. In the US research is increasing less than 10% each year. By the year 2020, or earlier, China will completely overtake the United States in medical research funding.

The information on astragalus in this text comes from three

main sources. First, original scientific research provides the vast majority of information written here. It is imperative that this large objective pool of scientific information becomes available to health professionals and non-scientists. Second, information from books, articles, and opinions of experts in herbal medicine are included. Third, information from my own experience utilizing astragalus with thousands of patients for over 30 years is also incorporated here.

INTRODUCTION

Paul was 1 1/2 years old when I first saw him. I spied him from my desk as his mom filled out the patient questionnaire form. He sat quietly with his head leaning against her. He looked tired, very tired, and so small and frail. I could see from 20 feet away this little guy was in trouble. When they came into the treatment room Paul's mom said, "You're my last hope." She told me how Paul was born prematurely and had developed normally in the first few months but then began to slow in his growth, falling significantly behind other children in his age group for weight and height. Pediatricians had diagnosed Paul with Failure to Thrive.

This general diagnosis is given to a child like Paul who, for some reason, is falling behind, significantly behind, other children in his age group. There are several reasons for Failure to Thrive: genetic errors of metabolism, digestive disorders, parental neglect, physical abuse, malnutrition, etc. Failure to Thrive is not as common in the United States as it is in poorer countries around the world. Paul's pediatrician had prescribed a pediatric multivitamin, as well as better nutrition with healthier food, but Paul was still suffering from poor development. This little guy was in deep trouble. His pediatrician recommended he be admitted to pediatric hospital care where he would receive IV nutrition and/or a feeding tube. Seeing the fear in the eyes of Paul's mom, I knew I had to do something that was acceptable to Paul, and that would work well and work quickly. This can be a difficult age to treat with herbs because patient compliance can be a big issue.

I knew what to do thanks not to teachers, research, or colleagues, but instead to a loving grandfather. Many years ago I was giving a lecture on medicinal plants of the Sierra Nevada, a specialty of mine, to a group of historians. An older gentleman came up to me afterwards and began to tell me about his granddaughter who had been diagnosed with Failure to Thrive and asked me if I knew anything about it. After a minute or two he pulled from his jacket a vial of Astragalus and said, "This is what cured my little granddaughter." Smiling, I said yes I know and have a strong affection for this plant. When I was sick with mono hepatitis as a young man, my recovery was incomplete until I drank a tea with astragalus as 25% of the formula. Ever since then I have researched astragalus, and prescribed it thousands of times alone or in combination with other herbs.

I prescribed astragalus liquid extract for Paul. After a few weeks a remarkable thing began to happen. Paul began to grow. He grew so fast and healthy that his pediatrician called me and said, and I will quote her here exactly, "I don't know how in the hell this works, but I want a case of it!" The treatment was simple, effective, and very impressive.

There are over 2,000 scientific studies on astragalus, and many give clues as to why astragalus is so effective for Failure to Thrive. Several studies have looked at how astragalus affects stem cell production. Numerous studies show that Astragalus enhances and transforms stem cells for bone growth, red blood cell and white blood cell proliferation. Many studies have also shown that astragalus has a highly significant action on boosting several immune functions.

While astragalus increases normal healthy cell growth, it also has been shown to turn off several types of cancer. This phenomenon, called apoptosis, is where cells die (turn off) without the toxic effects seen in typical chemotherapeutic or radiation induced necrosis. Apoptosis is the preferred way for cancer cells to die and some synthetic drugs and many natural plant chemicals (notably farnesol, geraniol, and limonene) are being studied to induce apoptosis in cancer cells. Astragalus has also been shown to increase the lifespan of normal cells. One of the latest areas of research is in the area of life extension. Astragalus has been shown to reduce the aging of telomeres, the protective caps on the ends of DNA strands that pass along genetic material. As we age telomeres begin to break down and shorten, but astragalus can help keep them intact and also keeps cells alive, delaying programmed cell death.

It is fascinating to think that a single plant can be so powerful and still have little or no side effects. Many herbs marketed as health building tonics have some major precautions, such as Chinese Ginseng and its stimulating quality. One contraindication for astragalus intake may (or may not) be for people who have received organ transplants and are taking immunosuppressive drugs such as cyclosporine and prednisone. Overwhelmingly astragalus actually helps many drugs work better. It has been shown to help Acyclovir's antiviral effects on herpes simplex, improve heart, liver, kidney and pancreas function, as well as enhance some chemotherapeutic medicines. Many more uses of this fascinating plant follow. Over the years I have used Astragalus in liquid, powder, capsules and whole roots for patients of all ages with a variety of health issues. It is exciting to think that an herb like this can be effective for both 11 month old children and 91 year old adults. I saw Paul again a few months ago. He is three now and looks and acts like any healthy youngster.

Chapter 1

WHAT IS ASTRAGALUS?

"That's it? That's astragalus? Not very impressive". That's what the botanical medicine student said as she stared at the astragalus bush near Lake Tahoe. I had to agree with her. Compared to the many beautiful wildflower laden plants of California, astragalus looks meek. But it's treasure is hidden from view. It's value to humans lies underground, in its roots. Astragalus is a small bush and a member of the pea family (Fabaceae) that grows throughout the world. There are over 400 different species of astragalus in North America alone. The Astragalus species that have been used for thousands of years are mainly *Astragalus membranaceus* and its subspecies *mongholicus*, neither of which grow in the United States. Presently botanists are considering changing the scientific name of both of these medicinal astragalus plants to *Astragalus pallidipurpeus*.[1] Astragalus membranaceus is also called *Astragalus propinquus*, which is the classification by the Russian botanist Boris Schischkin. The word astragalus means "vertebrae milk vetch". This refers to the leaf structure of the plant which has leaves opposite each other along stems, giving it a vertebrae-like appearance. There are several other medicinal astragalus species that grow in Asia and Europe. They are less well known and scantly researched compared to Astragalus membranaceus. Chinese medicinal astragalus is called Huang Qi (pronounced hwong chee) in the Mandarin dialect, meaning "yellow leader".

The first book to describe astragalus was the Chinese *Shennong Bencao Jing* written about one thousand years ago. In that text, astragalus is described as a medicine that treats infections, especially of the skin, improves deficient health, and treats hundreds of illnesses, especially in children. Since that time several books have described Astragalus as a tonic herb that helps defend against a broad range of illnesses. In traditional Chinese Medicine (TCM), astragalus is said to invigorate vital energy called qi (pronounced:chee). Qi is a fundamental concept in TCM. One of my early teachers, Harvard researcher Ted Kaptchuck, once wrote in his book, *The Web That Has No Weaver* that Qi "is matter on the verge of becoming energy, or energy at the point of materializing". Quantum physics may be one way of looking at qi, especially relating it to (super) string theory which states that energy at its most basic level can be seen in organized strings of vibrations. Are some of these strings of vibrations the meridians ancient Chinese physicians theorized 2000 years ago? Astragalus tonifies deficient qi of the lungs and digestive organs. It tonifies protective qi, called wei qi, assisting the body in defending against infections and environmental pollution. Many traditional Chinese medicine formulas have astragalus as an ingredient. Astragalus is quickly becoming the most popular Chinese medicinal herb in the world today.

It is the root of Astragalus that is used medicinally. The root itself can be shaped somewhat like a carrot, or more commonly can split several times as it's growing into multiple roots, and is usually sliced vertically or at a slight angle, sometimes resembling wooden tongue depressors. Wild roots, which are beginning to become scarce, are longer than cultivated roots and are generally less dense, especially in the outer layer of the root. Light yellow in color, the roots are also sold as powder, pills, teas, and prepared liquid drinks.

Astragalus is traditionally prepared by simmering in water to make tea or added to soups. Occasionally the roots are fried. The honey frying method became popular several hundred years ago. Traditionally honey frying astragalus is used by doctors of Chinese medicine to strengthen the digestive system and connective tissues of the body. Although simmering in water or soaking in alcohol extracts many chemicals in Astragalus, traditional honey-frying appears to damage some of the constituents and results in a lowering of antioxidant activity.[2,3]

There are many chemicals created within this plant that have a significant effect when isolated and used separately. As a whole root extract these chemicals work synergistically to make astragalus a very potent health promoting medicine. The three major components of astragalus are saponins, isoflavonoids, and polysaccharides.

The polysaccharides (starches) of astragalus are called astragalans. They are also referred to as APS (astragalus polysaccharides) and are non-caloric. They are mainly water soluble and are often extracted from the roots by cooking in water as a tea or added to soups. Some researchers have cooked astragalus in alcohol as well, extracting the polysaccharides without water.[4] Incredibly active chemicals, astragalus polysaccharides have been highly valued for their immune stimulating qualities and blood cell producing ability. They are also anti-inflammatory and antioxidant in nature. The amount of polysaccharides varies from plant to plant, with the range being between 10-20% of the entire root. Commercial astragalus extracts can have much higher amounts, up to 95% polysaccharides. Astragalus researchers are presently experimenting with methods to increase the level of polysaccharides in astragalus through fermentation with certain bacteria.[5]

Some researchers point out that a small amount of the starches found in astragalus are actually from bacteria that live in the root of this plant. Called bacterial endophytes, botanists believe that almost every plant in the world has these types of bacteria growing inside them. The bacteria do not hurt the plant, and are considered benign and harmless to people as well. If this theory is correct, and bacteria live inside every plant on earth, either in their roots, stems, leaves, flowers or seeds, it would mean that everyone, even vegetarians, are consuming from the animal kingdom.[6,7]

Next are the astragalus saponins. Most of the saponins are astragalosides. These sugar containing molecules are very active chemicals. Many scientific studies have utilized isolated astragalus saponins, especially astragaloside IV.[8-16] These chemicals are significantly effective in both preventing and repairing tissue damage from traumatic injury, increasing immune function, improving heart health, and reducing inflammation. They also exert a moderate antioxidant effect. Saponin content in the roots is usually about .1 to .2%, with some commercially available extracts of astragalus claiming to have up to 98% astragalus saponins. Wild astragalus roots contain more saponins than commercially grown plants.[17] Thin roots contain more astragalosides than thick roots.[18] Many astragalus researchers view astragaloside IV as the most interesting component of all those found in the roots of this plant. It is the astragalosides and their metabolite cycloastragenol that are concentrated into the anti-aging compound TA-65 that is mentioned in the life extension chapter. Adding other saponin containing herbs, such as ginseng or licorice, to astragalus formulas, greatly enhances the overall positive effects of these important chemicals.

Next are the flavonoids. Flavonoids are chemical compounds created within plants and act as antioxidant and stress response chemicals. The orange, red, and purple colors that appear in the leaves of many plants in autumn, for instance, are from flavonoids that help plants eek out a few more days of active status just before shutting down for winter. Most of these chemicals in astragalus are isoflavonoids. So far about 17 isoflavonoids have been discovered in the root of astragalus.[19-22] The yellow color of astragalus roots is due to the isoflavonoids. They are antioxidant, anti-inflammatory, increase the strength of tissue, and speed repair of injuries. Studies have shown that young astragalus roots have the same levels of isoflavonoids as older, thicker roots. Wild astragalus roots contain more isoflavonoids than cultivated plants.[23] Of all the isoflavonoid chemicals studied, calycosin appears to be the most potent antioxidant component.[24] Astragalus quality is often judged by its isoflavonoid content, with 0.5% of hydroxy-3-methoxy-isoflavone-7 being the minimal standard. These important chemicals are not in huge amounts in astragalus. To get the most effect from the isoflavonoids, a moderately large dose of astragalus is needed. Commercially available astragalus extracts can contain up to 4% isoflavonoids.

There are also minerals, mainly copper, iron, manganese, zinc, cobalt, and potassium, in astragalus.[25,26] There are traces of other chemicals as well. Amino acids, vitamin B3 (nicotinic acid), folic acid, vitamin B2 (riboflavin), as well as the fatty acids linoleic acid and alpha-linolenic acid are found in small amounts.[27,28] All in all, about six dozen chemical compounds have been isolated from astragalus. When buying sliced astragalus roots look for a light yellow color as a clue to the quality of astragalus roots.

Besides looking, one can smell for astragalus quality. A volatile chemical present in the root, called hexanal, produces a strong smoky sweet odor, called "beany flavor" in China. This pleasant odor correlates well with levels of polysaccharides and astragaloside IV. The stronger the beany flavor, the higher these important chemicals exist in astragalus.[29] If the smell of astragalus seems familiar, it is because hexanal is commonly used by food companies to create a fruity flavor in chewing gum and other processed foods.

In terms of cultivating astragalus, it is generally easy to grow. It's basically a hardy pea bush that withstands both dry and moderately humid environments. In damp environments it becomes susceptible to root and crown rot. This is one of the more perplexing challenges for cultivation of astragalus in China. To produce a more singular tap root, very loose, rich soil should be utilized. Otherwise much more splitting of the root occurs underground. Studies done on growing astragalus show that one could increase root polysaccharides by using a high potassium, medium phosphorus, and low nitrogen fertilizer. To increase astragalosides in astragalus root a high nitrogen, medium potassium, and low phosphorus fertilizer would be used. Flavonoid content is not altered by different fertilizer ratios.[30] It is a cold weather germinator, with early spring being optimal planting time. It is best to gently scrape (scarify) the seeds with fine sandpaper before planting to remove some of the hard coating of the seed. Inoculating astragalus seeds with rhizobium before planting greatly enhances the germination and health of the plants. I recommend Horizon Herb Company in Oregon for astragalus seeds.

There have been several studies on the safety of astragalus. None have found astragalus to be toxic to people, even at very high doses. Rarely, people with chronic headaches report that some astragalus-based formulas occasionally worsen them. By itself astragalus could rarely do this. Put into a formula that is strongly stimulating, such as with Chinese ginseng, astragalus could contribute to the worsening of some types of headaches. Other than this rare occurrence, it is safe for almost all people. Of course there is always the very slim chance that an individual could be allergic to one of the components of astragalus. I have rarely seen this occur. The one group of individuals that Astragalus may not be appropriate for would be those individuals who have undergone organ transplant surgery. The immune stimulating qualities of astragalus may (or may not) cause organ rejection. More on this later. Some people may experience loose stools or flatulence if they take a very large dose of Astragalus at one time. This is likely due to fermentation of the herb as it passes through the intestinal tract.

Astragalus does have anti-inflammatory and mild blood thinning qualities. These help prevent clot-type strokes and heart attacks. Astragalus has been shown to reduce excessive "stickiness" of blood cells. There are no reports that astragalus interacts adversely with typical anticoagulant drugs, which do not act through the same biological mechanisms as astragalus.[31] There was one study in the 1990's where astragalus, along with several other herbs, was reported to cause mutations in cells.[32] This study utilized what is called the Ames mutagenic test. This test is now largely discounted as a primary source of information because of its consistent unreliable nature. Many harmless chemicals, such as vitamin C, have been erroneously labeled mutagens with the Ames test. Recently, more sophisticated tests have found no mutagenic qualities for astragalus. In fact, they have found just the opposite. Astragalus actually prevents and can even reverse cellular mutations caused by synthetic chemicals.[33] Preventing and reversing mutations protects us from some very serious diseases such as cancer.

The ability of astragalus to increase or decrease a physiological response according to a patient's needs confound many health practitioners. Some see astragalus as only an inflammatory generating herb because it increases many immune functions that have inflammation as a part of a response to infection. Some think because astragalus is strongly anti-inflammatory against kidney disease and type 1 diabetes that it is only anti-inflammatory. There is even a popular protocol that prohibits astragalus from being used in chronic Lyme disease. The belief being that as the disease changes over time astragalus would not be helpful and would actually worsen the Lyme disease symptomatology. The idea being put forward is that astragalus only works in one direction and could not alter its effects to counteract the changing disease pattern. One of astragalus's best uses, however, is to do just that. It modifies disease in the direction of health. So far, there is no scientific data to back the chronic Lyme/astragalus prohibition.

Astragalus is called locoweed in the United States and some locoweed species can be very toxic. There are over 400 astragalus species in the United States. Some of these plants are hosts to a fungus called a fungal endophyte that grows on their leaves. This particular fungus produces a family of toxic chemicals called swainsonines.[34,35] Although early studies have shown anti-cancer activity for swainsonines, these chemicals are very toxic to the nervous system. When cattle or horses eat the fungus-contaminated leaves of locoweed when they graze, they become sick and often walk in a staggered gait which is called locoism.[36] The cattle look "loco" or crazy. The word locoweed has been used for hundreds of years. One of the first recorded uses of the word was by Captain Meriwether Lewis who wrote in his diary of encountering species of astragalus during the Lewis and Clark Expedition in 1802. He reported that native American tribes he encountered were well aware of locoweed's potential toxic effects with their horses. Fortunately, this toxic locoweed fungus does not grow on the roots of astragalus species that are used medicinally, so there is no chance of getting locoism from the medicinal astragalus varieties.

Some astragalus species are also what is called hyperaccumulators of the mineral selenium.[37] These particular species of astragalus grow in areas where large amounts of selenium exist in the soil. Plants growing there absorb and accumulate significant amounts of selenium. Although vital in small amounts in our diet to increase antioxidant activity and assist in thyroid function, selenium is toxic when eaten in moderate to large quantities, such as when cattle graze. The medicinal species of astragalus are not hyperaccumulators of selenium and are therefore safe. Interestingly, while hyperaccumulator species of astragalus grow robustly with high amounts of selenium in the soil, the medicinal species of astragalus actually grow very poorly in these types of soil.[38]

There has been much interest in the last twenty years in interactions between synthetic drugs and herbal medications. In many cases herbs effect how drugs are metabolized. Astragalus has been shown to slightly increase the time that some drugs remain active in our bodies.[39,40] So far, studies have shown that the interactions between astragalus and synthetic medications always benefit the patient. Astragalus often reduces drug toxicities and amplifies their positive benefits. Many drugs work better when astragalus is present. Astragalus has been shown to reduce toxic effects of several classes of drugs including immunosuppressants and paradoxically synthetic immune stimulators such as interleukin-2 (Il-2). This ability to improve drug actions while reducing side effects is a fascinating area that needs more research. If preliminary results of studies are correct and astragalus is continually shown to reduce toxicity and increase efficacy of many synthetic medications, one can see its use being increased simply as an aid to current drug therapies.

Recently, astragalus has become commercially available in very concentrated forms. This raises the possibility that an individual could consume hundreds or even thousands of times the amounts of the active ingredients found naturally in astragalus roots. Although no side effects of these research-level supplements have been reported, it is best to utilize these under supervision of a health professional who is well educated in astragalus use.

As the 1,000 year old Chinese *Shannong Bencao* herb book states, astragalus can treat many health problems. In the 21st century, astragalus is being utilized to prevent and treat a very large group of health problems. They include diabetes, cancer, immune deficiencies, heart disease, kidney disease, lung disease, infections, allergies, fractures and soft tissue injuries, brain injuries and strokes, radiation and chemotherapy effects, anemias of various causes, osteoporosis, inflammation, aging, failure to thrive syndrome, systemic lupus, liver disease including cirrhosis and hepatitis, stress syndromes, mental and physical exhaustion, environmental illness, etc. Astragalus can be used alone or in combination with other herbs and nutrients that augment and broaden astragalus's healing properties. In traditional Chinese medicine it is much more common to prescribe astragalus in combination with other herbs than just by itself.

There are over 2,000 studies on Astragalus that are either in original English or have been translated into English. As mentioned, most of these are from China, where the herb grows wild and is cultivated in great abundance. Scientists in other countries are also researching this plant as well, including the United States, Great Britain, Spain, France, New Zealand, Japan, South Korea, Croatia, Turkey, Taiwan, etc.

Chapter 2

ASTRAGALUS AND DIABETES

The pancreas is a vital organ that sits behind our stomach and liver. It has two main functions. First is its ability to produce digestive enzymes that are pushed into the upper small intestine to breakdown and digest food. Second, the pancreas controls blood sugar levels by creating insulin and glucagon. Insulin promotes entry of glucose into tissues, especially muscles, which lowers blood levels of this simple sugar. Glucagon promotes the breakdown of glycogen to glucose in the liver and other tissues which raises blood levels of sugar.

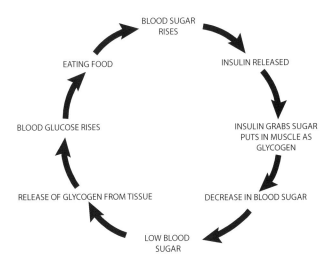

In healthy people, there is a balance of insulin and glucagon. In diabetes this balance is significantly abnormal. Type 1 diabetes, also called insulin dependent diabetes mellitus (IDDM), occurs when the immune system of an individual attacks and kills most to almost all of the cells in the pancreas that create insulin, called beta cells. Without healthy pancreatic beta cells producing insulin, an individual usually turns to daily insulin injections as maintenance for type 1 diabetes. Type 1diabetes usually occurs in childhood or early adolescence, in which case it is often referred to as juvenile diabetes. Adults do develop type 1 diabetes also. Often it occurs with adults after illness or stress, usually the combination of both. Type 1 diabetes is believed to result from genetic and environmental causes. There is a genetic influence on the development of Type 1 diabetes. Most people who have type one diabetes have an abnormality on their sixth chromosome. This is an inherited characteristic and may account for over 50% of insulin-dependent diabetes cases. This genetic influence also makes people susceptible to an environmental insult that triggers an autoimmune response.

This is a very important finding and represents one of the most underrated occurrences that affect people. That is that many diseases occur because there is a weakness genetically and then an insult environmentally. We all are born with dozens of mutations in our genetic code. Unless these mutations are stimulated and expressed by an environmental pollutant, virus, or other factors, most of those mutations will never harm us. Several studies have looked for a trigger for insulin dependent diabetes. Some show that a viral infection or early introduction to cow's milk can be the main insults in genetically susceptible people that trigger the body to begin a cascade of immune responses involving T lymphocytes and antibodies.[1-3] Viruses often have sequences of amino acids that are similar to pancreas amino acid sequences. This confuses the immune system and causes it to attack pancreas cells along with the virus.

The problem with cow's milk starts with the challenge that the lining of infant's intestines does not mature until the 6th to 7th month of life. Until that time, the intestines are very permeable. That is they have small holes in them that cannot keep large protein molecules from slipping through the intestinal wall and into the bloodstream. This causes an inflammatory response. This does not occur with human milk because our immune system recognizes this food as normal and non-foreign. Cow's milk is seen as a foreign non-self food and can cause a child's immune system to form antibodies to attack these milk proteins with tremendous force.

Casein, a major protein in both human and cow's milk, can cause a very significant antibody response that contributes to type one diabetes. The casein from cow's milk contains an important variant or difference in structure compared to human breast milk once it is digested. Unlike human milk casein, cow's milk casein can cause direct immune dysfunction and also has opioid properties. The casein content of cow's milk is four times more than human milk. Bovine Serum Albumin(BSA), another protein in cow's milk, also shows cross reactivity that can cause autoimmune responses against the pancreas.

Besides the BSA problem, Cow's milk also has a surface protein similar to one in the pancreas called GAD (glutamic acid decarboxylase). The amino acid glutamic acid is converted in the pancreas via GAD into a neurotransmitter called GABA (gamma amino butyrate). GABA is used by the pancreas as a signaling molecule between pancreatic islets, the small glands that secrete insulin. Once the immune system targets cow's milk casein proteins, it also targets these similar proteins in the pancreas. Although the pancreas is an innocent bystander, this similarity of GAD proteins causes the body to mistakenly attack the pancreas after the cow's milk proteins have created an immune response. GAD antibodies can also occur in children developing diabetes who do not have cow's milk in their diet. Early introduction to cereal grains can also cause autoimmunity in some infants, especially those grains that contain gluten. Whatever the cause or combination of causes, this inflammatory response is what is responsible for the immune system killing pancreas cells.

There is, and has been for several decades, a heated debate among pediatric researchers as to the question if young children should be given cow's milk at all. Right now the general consensus is that cow's milk should not be given to any child less than one year of age. Some physicians believe that cow's milk is poorly digested by a large percentage of older children and adults as well. Noted biochemist, Thomas Campbell, who co-authored the largest study ever conducted on nutrition, the Cornell China study, states,

"Cow's milk may cause one of the most devastating diseases that can befall a child, Type 1 diabetes."[4]

Over 75% of people who have type 1 diabetes have antibodies to their own pancreatic beta cells. Only about 1% of non-diabetic Americans have these antibodies. Some researchers believe that certain viruses themselves damage beta cells directly.[5] There is little or no repair of any of this pancreatic damage in Type 1 diabetes with synthetic medications.[6]

Type 2 diabetes is also known as non-insulin dependent diabetes mellitus (NIDDM). Over 90% of all diabetics have this type. Type 2 diabetes is often a self-inflicted disease, preventable with proper diet, exercise, and weight reduction. In 1996, 15 million Americans struggled with diabetes. Today (2014) almost 10 percent (30 million Americans) now have either insulin dependent or non-insulin dependent diabetes. The almost doubling of this disease in less than 20 years, and the fact that worldwide over 250 million people have diabetes, understates that this is the biggest health problem that faces modern society. In non-insulin diabetes, the five main causes are: 1) lack of exercise, 2) destructive eating habits, consuming too much processed nutrient-deficient food, and too much sugar specifically, 3) becoming overweight because of poor eating and lethargy, 4) genetic predisposition to diabetes, 5) environmental insult leading to pancreatic autoimmunity.

There is also latent autoimmune diabetes (LADA) which is similar to type one diabetes, in that GAD antibodies attack pancreatic cells. But in LADA the damage is very slow and often does not appear until adulthood. This type of diabetes is under diagnosed and under treated. Testing for GAD antibodies would help predict LADA and type 1 diabetes.

According to studies at the United States Department of Agriculture, the average person in the United States now eats over 150 pounds of sugar per year. This translates to over 42 teaspoonfuls of sugar per day. This is a significant difference from what humans ate up until about one hundred years ago. Just in the last 50 years our average sugar intake has increased over 50%. In 1960 the average

American's intake of high fructose corn syrup was just a few ounces per year. Today it is over 2,000 ounces (65 pounds).[7] Over 99% of the time Homo sapiens have been evolving, survival depended on successful hunting and gathering of wild food. Agriculture didn't take hold until about 10,000 years ago. Even then it was unusual for people to eat grains that were stripped of their fiber and devoid of the nutrients held in the fiber and germ of the plant. That leaves 300,000 plus years of evolving with very little sugar in the diet. With the exception of honey, there were few concentrated sources of sugar other than wild fruits. These ancient wild fruits such as strawberries, kumquats, bilberries, choke cherries, and grapes also contained the fiber, minerals, vitamins, and other chemicals that helped metabolize their sugar.[8-11]

Today our diets are far different from our ancestors. A large portion of the human race is now participating in a worldwide experiment to see of we can survive this dramatic increase in sugar, processed foods, and obesity. At present we are failing that experiment. Almost one in three Americans are obese. Over 90% of all people who have type 2 diabetes are obese. We are now experiencing exactly the opposite of what our species experienced 100,000 years ago. That is, in ancient times humans struggled to gain weight. Weight loss was a condition of starvation from lack of food. Today many people struggle to lose weight. Now, weight gain is a condition of eating too much easily available processed foods high in sugar. A recent Center For Disease Control chart comparing restaurant portion sizes of 50 years ago versus today shows that the average meal served is 300% to 600% bigger now than it was in 1960.[12] **See chart**.

In terms of fat intake, our diets have also changed dramatically in the last few thousand years. Not much is said about how different dietary fats are today than a century ago. There was very little use of highly processed plant oils until the 1920's. Before that time, oils were pressed by small companies or family owned flax or olive producers. In Europe it was common to have an oil press that was village owned with the seeds or olives supplied by the local growers.

The oils were extremely fresh and pure. That has changed. The nutritional challenge now is to eat fats that are fresh (non-rancid), and not altered by heat and light. Fats that are hydrogenated or partially hydrogenated are not metabolized correctly, and instead cause significant amounts of inflammation.

FOOD PORTIONS 1950s TO NOW

Our bodies are designed to eat foods high in unaltered essential fatty acids, found in wild seeds and nuts, fish such as salmon, and wild meats such as venison. Eating these lowers the chance of developing type 2 diabetes. Eating highly processed agriculture grown oils (omega-6), such as safflower, sunflower, corn, etc., can increase that risk if those polyunsaturated oils are overcooked.

Cooking these polyunsaturated oils at high heat warps their molecular structure, causing them to increase cellular mutations and create inflammatory prostaglandin chemicals within our bodies. Commercial non-organic oils are processed through about a dozen steps that strip them of vitamins, minerals, and other natural compounds that protect the oils from rancidity. This is done to reduce the taste of the oils. Many vegetable oil companies strive for a light colored, bland tasting oil that they believe customers want. As bad as overheating these oils is, sunlight and even normal lighting in stores and at home can age polyunsaturated oils rapidly as well. If possible, buy oils in dark green or brown bottles that reduce light exposure to the fragile oils.

To complicate matters even more, people who have diabetes, especially type 1, have a reduced capacity to create anti-inflammatory chemicals from omega-6 oils. This is not an isolated challenge for diabetics. Other nutritional metabolic inefficiencies also take place in diabetes, including a serious reduction in the ability to create Vitamin A from carotenes in plants.

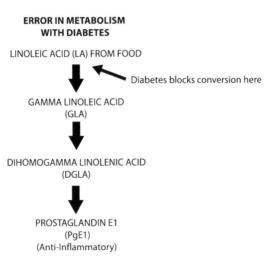

As a society we are consuming a diet that our bodies are not designed to eat. This is creating the immune and inflammatory disease we call diabetes. Imagine an assembly line that suddenly has parts that don't fit moving down the line. That is what is happening to people consuming large amounts of sugary processed foods. At that level sugar becomes not a food but instead a poison with major consequences of multiple diseases and premature death.

Diabetes starts slowly and silently. Symptoms appear not at the beginning of disease but begin several years after subtle changes start happening in the biochemistry and cells of future diabetics. By the time symptoms appear, most people are far along in this disease.

For those individuals with early or advanced diabetes, much can be done to reverse the terrible problems that evolve with his disease. Over 100 studies have confirmed that astragalus is very potent in improving diabetes for the vast number of people who utilize this as a primary or adjunctive anti-diabetic medicine. Unlike synthetic diabetic drugs, which only lower blood sugar, astragalus can improve most of the challenges diabetics face including high blood sugar levels, diabetic induced nephropathy (kidney disease), heart disease, immune deficiencies, inflammation, premature aging, fatigue, poor wound healing, peripheral neuropathy (numbness, tingling, and pain in the hands and/or feet), and retinopathy.

Mary T., a 35 year old bank executive, is talking on the phone to a customer when she begins to feel light headed. Even after taking a break she can't shake the feeling of fatigue, dizziness, and a mild aching in her lower back. Told by her doctor several months ago that she had high blood sugar levels in her latest blood test, Mary thought she had everything under control. She ate a little less sugar and felt that this alone would help her enough to keep her blood sugar under control. But what Mary didn't know was that deep inside her body, excess sugar was causing a profound inflammatory immune response. Blood glucose was attaching to the walls of her kidney cells and causing damage to the filtering system of her blood. Her kidney function was beginning to decline as her kidney cells became inefficient. Those cells were being attacked by her own immune system and began to die. A lab test, called the glomerular filtration rate estimate or GFRe, revealed that Mary's kidneys were only operating at 30% capacity. She had full blown kidney disease (nephropathy), and was on her way to serious kidney failure and dialysis.

About one-third to one-half of all diabetics develop nephropathy.[13] Her blood sugar levels were peaking at 70%-90% above normal. Shaken out of her comfort zone, Mary turned to traditional Chinese medicine to help her. Astragalus was prescribed as a single medicine for her diabetes and its ensuing kidney disease. She was also encouraged to begin switching her food intake away from large intakes of dairy and meat instead to a more plant-based diet. This reduces protein levels, which are usually too high in most diets, and increases nutrient intake since vegetables are generally high in healthful nutrients. Eating large amounts of foods that are high in animal protein causes the kidneys to work harder to filter out protein-containing nitrogen from the blood. Adding more work for the kidneys at the same time they are getting the tar beaten out of them by diabetes is not a good idea. The important thing in reduction of proteins is to not substitute starches like flour for them. Eating more vegetables and salads should be the goal.

Within two weeks Mary began feeling better and in two months her physician was astonished at Mary's new lab report. Her blood sugar was down, her energy was up, and most significantly, her kidney filtering function had improved from 30% to 50%. This could only mean her kidneys had not only stopped worsening but actually began to rejuvenate. Continual therapy after one year of her taking astragalus resulted in her kidney function improving to 70%. Her blood glucose was now near normal and Mary reported that she felt better then she had for a long time.

It's important to remember that diabetes takes several years to develop. During its development there is a large inflammatory response involving chemicals called cytokines. Cytokines are small proteins produced by many cells, including immune cells. They are grouped in several classes that include: interleukins, tumor necrosis factors, interferons, colony-stimulating factors, transforming growth factors, and chemokines. Many of these chemicals are responsible for the chronic and harmful inflammatory responses that drive the destruction of kidney tissue in diabetic nephropathy.[14,15] Astragalus has been shown to protect and repair kidneys in several important ways, including altering cytokine production. Studies on astragalus reveal its strong antioxidant and anti-inflammatory effects on kidney tissue, protecting it from further damage. Inflammatory chemicals called NF-KappaB are reduced by astragalus, blood lipids are more efficiently metabolized, blood sugar levels are reduced, and the rate in which kidneys repair is significantly increased.

In their analysis of 1804 patients (945 treated with astragalus and 859 used as controls), Dr. Li and his colleagues at the China Huashan Hospital's Department of Nephrology, found that astragalus significantly improved kidney laboratory scores of BUN, SCr, CCr, urine protein, and serum albumin.[16] These positive test results point to astragalus' ability to enhance kidney function and repair.

In their review of the kidney protective effects of astragalus, Dr. Zhang and his fellow researchers at the West China Hospital Department of Nephrology looked at 13 animal trials and found that astragalus reduced blood sugar levels and significantly improved kidney filtering capacity in all of them.[17] A study on how astragalus helps diabetic kidney disease found that astragalus protects kidneys through several multiple pathways at the gene level.[18] Astragalus affects several hundred genes in our bodies.

In 2007 researchers studied lab rats who had full blown diabetes-caused kidney disease. The rats had dull bristly hair and rapidly deteriorating muscles. Their spines began to age rapidly leading to a rounding of their skeleton called kyphosis. Their blood fat levels were abnormally high, they had sores that would not heal, and they were lethargic and exhausted easily. The animals blood sugar levels were very high, and inflammatory chemicals inside the kidneys were slowly destroying their function. These are the exact same things that happen in people with diabetes. By simply adding an astragalus tea to the lab animal's water supply, researchers found that all of the above serious signs and symptoms improved dramatically.[19] Astragalus caused a remarkable rejuvenation of kidney cells.

Creating more blood vessels to nourish damaged kidney tissue is an astragalus strong point. This blood vessel creation is called angiogenesis. In angiogenisis new blood vessels sprout or split from preexisting blood vessels. As we will see later in this text, astragalus also strongly promotes angiogenesis for wound repair. Getting new blood vessels to grow in damaged tissue is a key to rapid healing. People with diabetes have poor angiogenesis in general and really respond to the blood vessel creation action of astragalus. Astonishingly, in cases of cancer, astragalus actually does the opposite, reducing angiogenesis to tumor cells, which starves them by cutting off their nutrient supply. This example illustrates the many times where astragalus increases a chemical compound in one situation and reduces production in another. This ability to change or modulate body functions in the direction of health is why astragalus should be known as an alterative.

Not to be confused with the word alternative, alteratives promote health by altering chemical reactions and body functions to move in the direction of health. For example, astragalus can mildly reduce high blood pressure in people with hypertension, and can raise blood pressure in people who have abnormally low blood pressure (hypotension). This concept is a real challenge for many medical doctors to accept, as very few (none?) synthetic drugs are alteratives. For example, if a synthetic blood pressure medication is taken to reduce hypertension, blood pressure is hopefully reduced and taking more of the drug will only continue to push blood pressure down. Astragalus's ability to modulate or push blood pressure in the direction that is healthier regardless if blood pressure is too high or too low is very different. Another interesting fact is that if a person, who has no blood pressure problems, takes astragalus there is no affect at all on their blood pressure. This is accomplished by astragalus' ability to affect hundreds of genes that rule homeostatic (balancing) functions in our bodies. For example, genes that promote inflammation, needed in acute injury, and genes that reduce inflammation are both affected by astragalus, but only in the appropriate situations, and only when needed. Astragalus upregulates genes (expression) or downregulates genes (suppression) based on the specific need at that moment in that particular area of the body.

Besides kidney damage, diabetes also accelerates heart disease. Diabetes causes a significant rise in inflammation and increases fat in our bloodstream. Large amounts of oxidation will occur. Oxidation, here being the stealing of electrons from atoms of the lining of arteries called the endothelium, is the genesis of atherosclerosis. The heart muscle itself can then become damaged and inefficient, and cardiomyopathy results. Cardiomyopathy is any abnormality of the structure and function of the heart and its vessels. About a dozen studies have utilized astragalus in diabetic-induced cardiomyopathy. All of them show that astragalus reverses the inflammatory and oxidative states in diabetic cardiomyopathy. There are about two dozen damaging chemicals that are generated in this disease. Astragalus reduces these toxic chemicals and increases healing chemicals in the heart.[20-24]

The immune system in diabetics is slow, not very bright, and very weak. Studies have shown that even in people who do not have diabetes, drinking the equivalent of two sodas (18-22 teaspoons of sugar) causes a significant sluggishness of macrophages. These immune cells either do not recognize bacteria at all or when these white blood cells do recognize foreign bacteria, they move sluggishly toward the bacteria and are much less powerful against the invasive organisms. It takes several hours for the immune system to return to normal after a large dose of liquid sugar is consumed.[25]

Actually it is worse in diabetes, especially type one. The immune system goes berserk. While the diabetic immune system becomes inefficient at defending against infections, it instead begins to destroy pancreatic cells called beta cells. Beta cells produce insulin. In insulin dependent diabetes this immune dysfunction happens much more quickly with more devastating consequences than in non-insulin dependent diabetes. It's insulin's job to attach to sugar and present it to the body for normal metabolism. When blood sugar levels stay chronically high, immune cells called CD8 T cells begin to be produced in high numbers. The CD8 T cells then move to the pancreas and begin to bombard it with toxic chemicals. This slowly destroys the pancreatic function of producing insulin and lowering blood sugar. Astragalus turns off the overproduction of CD8 T cells, and protects the delicate insulin producing beta cells.[26] Astragalus significantly normalizes immune function in those individuals with diabetes.[27-29]

People with diabetes produce toxic chemicals called advanced glycation end products (AGEs). Many of these chemicals are responsible for the development of diabetic complications such as eye disease (retinopathy) and kidney disease (nephropathy). AGEs also damage the cells that line the inside of our arteries, called the endothelium. Once the endothelium is damaged, the process of atherosclerosis begins in earnest. AGEs cause the cells that line the kidneys to die. They also induce a type of kidney cell called a mesangial cell to proliferate far beyond its normal amount, which reduces kidney filtering ability and causes a dangerous increase in nitrogen compounds in the bloodstream. In a 2011 study at the Macau University of Science and Technology, astragalus isoflavonoids were used to determine if AGEs-induced kidney damage could be reduced. In this study astragalus was able to stop kidney cell death and normalize the cells that line kidney tissue.[30]

Macrophages are immune cells that usually help us by attacking foreign substances like viruses. It is important to remember that in non-insulin dependent diabetes our bodies become so poisoned by poor lifestyle choices that we are not recognized by the immune system as being normal humans. Instead, we are recognized as foreign objects to be attacked. Upon gaining entrance into kidney tissue that is inflamed, macrophages attack and destroy the kidney membranes. Researchers at the State Key Laboratory of Quality Research in Chinese Medicine set up a study to see if astragalus could reduce this infiltration of macrophages into diabetes-induced inflamed kidney tissue. Results of the study showed that astragalus significantly reduced macrophage migration and destruction. Researchers could actually witness this reduction in kidney inflammation and cell death at the molecular genetic level.[31] A similar study at the Shanghai Fifth Peoples Hospital in Fudan China found that astragalus inhibits AGEs inflammation by macrophages by redirecting them genetically to power down and stop attacking human cells.[32]

As wonderful as these results are, it would be best to prevent the early formation of these toxic AGEs. Could astragalus prevent their creation? Researchers at the Graduate School of Medical and Pharmaceutical Sciences in Japan fed diabetic mice an extract of astragalus and measured the production of AGEs. They found that astragalus inhibited AGEs production. Further study on their part revealed that it was the astragalosides in astragalus that were the most potent anti-AGEs compounds.[33]

Although many of the early signs of diabetes and its complications go unnoticed at first, there is a complication of diabetes that people really do notice. The body does not heal very well any more. Even small cuts are easily infected, and often take weeks or even months to heal. That healing is often of very poor quality, producing scar tissue in place of what was once normal healthy skin. The feet get the worst of it due to several factors including poor circulation. Often ulcers develop and infection sets in. Diabetics are 25 times more likely to have a leg amputated because of non-healing foot ulcers.[34] Several studies have investigated whether astragalus could help with wound healing, especially foot ulcers, in diabetics. Astragalus, alone or as an ingredient in several Chinese herbal formulas, has been shown to increase the speed in which ulcers heal, increasing blood vessel production in the damaged area.[35,36] Astragalus reduces ulcer scarring, and induces a very strong anti-inflammatory action. The most active anti-inflammatory ulcer healing ingredient of astragalus appears to be the flavonoid formononetin.[37] This is due to formononetin's ability to act as very strong suppressor of toxic nitrogen free radical chemicals in the wound area that normally would increase tissue damage.[38] Astragaloside IV is also a main player in ulcerative wound healing. This natural astragalus compound enhances protein proliferation and wound healing via its ability to turn on tissue repairing genes.[39] In a fascinating series of studies performed by scientists at the City University of Hong Kong, researchers checked 10,000 human genes to find the specific molecular mechanisms responsible for repair of diabetic ulcers by a combination of astragalus with the root of the Chinese plant rehmanniae. They found that a 2:1 ratio of astragalus to rehmanniae caused the expression of 116 genes responsible for cell proliferation, blood vessel growth (angiogenesis), and tissue repair.[40]

In most people struggling with non-insulin dependent diabetes, they begin to develop a resistance to insulin. Insulin begins to not work as efficiently, and some people develop antibodies to insulin itself. Many researchers point to insulin resistance as a key component for the etiology of non-insulin dependent diabetes. Several studies show that astragalus increases the efficiency of insulin, and decreases insulin resistance.[41-44] Genetic studies at the Beijing University of Chinese Medicine showed that a mixture of astragalus and the herb potentilla discolor causes a genetic expression of several genes that reduce insulin resistance.[45]

One of the more common problems with advanced diabetes is peripheral neuropathy. The insulating lining of nerves, called myelin, begins to be destroyed by white blood cells. White blood cells move to the sugar-poisoned myelin and spit oxidative chemicals that cause the myelin to break down. With the nerve insulation damaged, nerve fibers become exposed and inflamed, and tingling, pain, and numbness begins. Most commonly seen in the feet, neuropathy can be very debilitating. Astragalus offers tremendous assistance in reversing this diabetic disease. It has been shown to repair and replace damaged myelin through several molecular mechanisms.[46]

Another major problem with diabetes is its effects on vision. The retina, the posterior portion of the eye that allows us to see clearly, is dramatically damaged by inflammatory responses to high levels of blood sugar. Cells known as pericytes or mural cells, which normally protect the cells lining retinal capillaries, begin to die from the accumulation of sorbitol (an alcohol sugar) and advanced glycation end products.[47] Called diabetic retinopathy, people begin to lose their frontal vision and the condition usually continues until the person is almost totally blind except for extreme peripheral vision.

In a recent review of 16 clinical trials of astragalus and its effects on diabetic retinopathy, researchers report that astragalus improved visual acuity and enhanced general eye health. The researchers cautioned that these findings are early and are of low methodological quality.[48] In a very interesting animal trial with the addition of panax notoginseng (Tian Qi) to the astragalus-angelica sinensis combination known as Dang Gui Bu Xue Tang, rats with diabetic retinopathy were given this combination with dramatic results. This astragalus combination prevented the progression of retinopathy. Sophisticated measurements of inflammatory chemicals found that these herbs decreased the expression of inflammatory interleukins, tumor necrosis factor alpha, NF-kappaB, and several other retinopathy inducing chemicals.[49]

Astragalus is an effective non-toxic medical intervention for both type 1 and type 2 diabetes. It is not, however, a substitute for a healthy lifestyle. The ability for any medical intervention to successfully assist in improving a persons health is limited by lifestyle choices, and whether they are healthy or destructive. In the 21st century we will see if Americans, and indeed the world population, are up to the task of making good lifestyle choices. As good as astragalus is in helping the body be more efficient and healthier, it cannot do it alone. It really is difficult to save a person from themselves. I often tell my patients that I am somewhat like the Marines. That is, I am looking for a few good patients. Patients that want to thrive, not just survive. There is some room for optimism in that obesity rates that drive type-2 diabetes in the United States are stabilizing for the first time in 40 years. A significant drop (about 43%) in childhood obesity was reported by the Centers for Disease Control in 2014.

Chapter 3

ASTRAGALUS AND IMMUNITY

Our immune system is a very complex combination of cells. It's a community of cells really. That community of cells communicates with each other and responds to anything deemed as non-self or foreign, as well as any substance it views as dangerous. Over the last ten years a tremendous amount of research has been done on immune cells and the chemicals they produce.

If a person is familiar with astragalus it is often in the context that they have heard that astragalus helps immunity. There are over 100 scientific studies on astragalus' effect on immune function. Actually, if we include studies in cancer and other diseases that are governed by immune function the amount is over 300 studies. For hundreds of years doctors have seen astragalus work in clinical practice, but in the 21st century we also want to know how it does what it does. Fortunately, modern research has now shown how astragalus affects our immune system at the molecular level. Researchers can now see how astragalus works. And work it does. In a bacterial infection for example, astragalus increases the body's response against the bacteria. White blood cells are created faster, recognize the bacteria quicker, move towards it faster, and kill it quicker with much more powerful effects. Our white blood cells spit very toxic oxidant free radical chemicals (super oxide, hydrogen peroxides, singlet oxygen, etc) at the bacteria while at the same time protecting themselves with antioxidant chemicals. Astragalus enhances these actions dramatically.[1-5]

Perhaps astragalus' best immune effect is in preventing infections. In traditional Chinese medicine (TCM), preventing disease by assisting in patients good health is the premier goal. Preventive medicine has been a hallmark of TCM for over 2000 years. As a person takes astragalus over several days or weeks, the immune system is nourished to be smarter, stronger, and much more efficient. One of the most effective uses of Astragalus clinically is in people who chronically get bacterial or viral infections. It is not normal to get several colds and/or influenza every year. Astragalus can be a great preventive for these people. I have had many patients take astragalus in this situation with dramatic improvements. I once treated an Olympic wrestler who, although he looked healthy, consistently came down with bronchitis and subsequent pneumonia nearly every winter. I prescribed moderately large doses of astragalus for him to take every day in both tea and pill form. He never had bronchitis/pneumonia again.

One myth about astragalus is that it will cause acute viral infections to worsen, especially herpes viruses and varicella (chicken pox/shingles). There is absolutely no data to support this absurd claim. The truth is that astragalus directly enhances immune function to eliminate viral infections and greatly increases the effectiveness of many, if not all, anti-viral medicines.

If there is any toxicity or inappropriate use of astragalus it may be with individuals who have transplanted tissue in their bodies. Immunosuppressive drugs that prevent the transplant recipient from rejecting the transplanted foreign organ do so by lowering immunity in that person. Astragalus has been shown to reverse immune suppression and that action may theoretically cause organ rejection. Many health care practitioners believe that because astragalus increases immune function, it would also cause a rejection of transplanted tissue. There are few examples of this either way. In the two studies that actually looked at astragalus' effect on transplantation, the opposite occurred. Allographs are transplanted tissue within the same species who are not related genetically. In an experiment to see if transplanting allograph blood vessels from one strain of mice into another type of mice would be rejected as normally expected, scientists observed that the mice who did not receive astragalus showed white blood cells attacking and rejecting the transplanted arteries. In the astragalus group there was no immune system attack. Astragalus prevented the inflammatory immune response that would have caused tissue rejection.[6]

In a more recent Japanese study on allograph survival, mice

receiving transplants showed no difference in rejection between an astragalus group and an immunosuppressed group who were given cyclosporine. Sophisticated investigation of the molecular mechanisms responsible for this anti-rejection effect showed that astragalus reduced the genetic expression of inflammatory genes.[7] More research is needed, but these are very interesting early findings.

Organ transplant is one of the three situations that astragalus intake may be contraindicated. One other is during high fever due to infection. Some natural health care practitioners are concerned that astragalus may drive fever higher in what is called a cytokine storm, where the immune system gets too revved up for our own good, and drives fever to dangerous levels. However, there is no scientific evidence that cytokine storms caused by astragalus actually occur. In fact, astragalus does not enhance the type of cytokines, called IL-1beta, that cause inflammation and high fevers. It appears that the opposite is true. Researchers at the University of Texas-Houston Medical School found that astragalus reduces pro-inflammatory fever responses that occur during infection.[8] Astragalus also inhibits Tumor Necrosis Factor which is the other main cause of fevers.

Lastly, simply because not enough studies have been done with pregnant women and astragalus, it is advised not to take astragalus during pregnancy. There was one study on pregnant rats and rabbits that showed that astragaloside IV caused fetal death and toxicity to the rats in the study. Upon close examination, the human equivalent of the doses used in the experiment was over 720,000 milligrams of astragalus. For people, that would be about two and one-half pounds of astragalus each dose. This would be impossible to achieve in humans.

Astragalus has been broadly researched and clinically utilized in a variety of immune diseases and illnesses. Astragalus has been shown to reduce herpes simplex 1 infection and multiplication, prevent toxoplasmosis infection, increase the effectiveness of HIV antiviral drugs, prevent and cure cytomegalovirus infections, cure systemic candidiasis (yeast infections), reduce infection, speed repair after tissue injury, improve immune function in myasthenia gravis patients, prevent cryptosporidium infection, increase immunity in individuals with poor immune function, increase white blood cell and red blood cell counts to normal, and reduce infections and organ damage in autoimmune diseases such as lupus.[9-13] As we will see in the chapter on cancer, astragalus reduces the immune suppressing effects of chemotherapy and radiation therapy as well.

The research on myasthenia gravis is especially interesting. This is an autoimmune disease where the body creates antibodies to its own acetylcholine receptors. These nervous system receptors control our ability to move. Damaging them causes significant muscle weakness and fatigue, especially in the eye muscles. Utilizing astragalus for this disease may surprise even the most experienced herbalists who may believe that astragalus, being an immune stimulant, would feed the autoimmune response and worsen this disease. The exact opposite occurred when 60 myasthenia gravis patients were studied in this astragalus experiment. Thirty patients were given prednisone and thirty patients were given astragalus. Prednisone is an effective immune system suppressor with significant side effects when delivered at large dosages for several weeks or longer. In the experiment both prednisone and astragalus reduced inflammation and the overproduction of white blood cells. Astragalus did not increase an abnormal immune response, but instead reduced the autoimmune response just as effectively as prednisone. Perhaps the most important safety finding was that in the prednisone group five patients experienced temporary liver damage. There was no liver damage, or any other side effect, with the astragalus group.[14]

Almost everyone in the U.S., at one time or another, is checked with the tuberculin skin test to make certain they are not infected with tuberculosis (TB). In this terrible disease, lung tissue is slowly destroyed by TB organisms. Other organs can be infected as well, such as the brain, kidneys, liver, etc. When a person is infected with tuberculosis, the first major response is from immune cells called macrophages. It is macrophages job to recognize and signal an attack on tuberculosis. If macrophages are too few in number or sluggish and weak in their action, tuberculosis will increase its invasion into our bodies and require serious medication for its cure. Health care workers who specialize in TB treatment must have efficient immune function to ward off this disease. Scientists studying TB at Lanzhou University in China found that astragalus significantly increases the power of macrophages to attack and destroy the mycobacterium that causes tuberculosis.[15]

Over the last thirty years the world has seen an epidemic of Human Immunodeficiency Virus (HIV). HIV hijacks immune cells known as CD4 cells. The virus enters the CD4 cell and uses the cell as a breeding ground for itself. This kills the CD4 cell in the process, thereby severely lowering immune function. Other immune cells are also killed, including dendritic cells and macrophages. Over the last three decades, scientists have been developing drugs to combat HIV infection. Many countries are struggling to deliver medicine to infected people to extend their lives. HIV medicines, called retrovirals, are expensive. Many people in the world infected with this disease cannot afford these medications. The current drug strategy is to combine two to three drugs together to give HIV infected people the best chance of living a longer life. Researchers throughout the world are working on finding a cure for HIV infection.

Research with astragalus and HIV began in 2004, when a study utilizing astragalus in a combination medicine showed reduction of HIV infection by up to 35%.[16] In a gold standard study (randomized, double blind, placebo-controlled) from the Thailand Ministry of Health, HIV-positive people were given either a standard two drug combination (ZVD and ddC) combined with a placebo, or the same two antiviral drugs plus an astragalus-based herbal combination. Their findings were impressive. While the two antiviral/placebo combination did moderately lower the levels of HIV in the patients blood stream and increased CD4 cells, it was the astragalus combination that significantly lowered HIV count in 4 weeks and continued to increase the number of CD4 cells far better than in the two drug/placebo group. This study lasted for 6 months, and left researchers with the opinion that astragalus could be very helpful and much less expensive than adding a third synthetic drug to anti-HIV regimens.[17]

Our thymus gland, which sits on top of our heart and lungs, produces immune cells called T lymphocytes (the "T" comes from the word thymus), especially when we are young. It reaches maximum size just before puberty. Sex hormones created during puberty signal the thymus to shrink. It continues shrinking as we age. The thymus weighs about an ounce at age ten and is about half that weight when we are about fifty. By the time we are in our seventies it is only about a quarter ounce in weight. Stem cells (thymocytes) are sent from the bone marrow to the thymus where they mature into T-cells. T-cells are extremely important for proper immune function. For example, one of the main reasons elderly people are more susceptible to infection is their reduced thymus size and activity. Fortunately, we create a large storage of T-cells early in life that continue to reproduce themselves for many years. T-cells help the body recognize foreign invaders such as viruses. This ability for T-cells to distinguish between normal tissue and foreign invading microbes enables us to properly fight infection. An interesting study at the Shantou University Medical College in China found that Astragalus could increase the size of the thymus gland, and improve its ability to create T- cells, even after it was insulted with the immune suppressing drug cyclophosphamide (Cytoxin). An even better thymus-stimulating effect was found when astragalus was combined with the herb he shou wu (*Polygonum multiflorum/ Reynoutria multiflora*).[18]

Astragalus is a powerful immune system modulator. It has been shown to increase specific immune responses to multiple diseases as well as alter immune function to reduce immune response when that benefits the patient. Either alone or in combination with other herbs, astragalus offers an opportunity to live a healthier life with fewer infections and immune diseases.

Chapter 4

ANEMIA AND LEUKOPENIA

There are over two dozen types of anemia, which is a reduction in red blood cells. Red blood cells are made in the bone marrow of our long bones and, once expressed out into the blood stream, mature and live about 120 days. Red blood cells carry oxygen to our tissues, nourishing them every second of our lives. Anemias occur due to many causes that include: blood loss through injury or disease, nutritional deficiencies, genetic tendencies, kidney or thyroid disease, immune disease, etc. Astragalus can dramatically increase the production of erythropoietin (EPO), the kidney factor that turns on bone marrow to make more red blood stem cells. **SEE Box.**

THE EPO STORY

1. **Low oxygen levels in bloodstream are detected.**

2. **The outer portion of the kidneys, called the renal cortex, begins to produce EPO.**

3. **The EPO circulates in the bloodstream and finds and binds to receptors on red blood progenitor (stem-like) cells surface.**

4. **This activates chemical signals that cause red blood cells to mature and increase in numbers.**

Several studies have shown that astragalus, alone or with other herbs, induces a critical regulator called hypoxia response element (HRE), as well as increasing the expression of hypoxia-inducible factor (HIF) to promote EPO production at the genetic level.[1-3] You may have heard of EPO in the last ten years because some athletes, such as competitive cyclists, inject EPO into their bodies to make more red blood cells in an attempt to increase their blood cell oxygen levels and athletic performance. The ability of astragalus to stimulate red blood production has encouraged many research projects. All of these studies have found astragalus very helpful in reversing anemia without side effects.[4-7]

White blood cells, called leukocytes, are immune cells. They guard our bodies against infection and cancer. Leukopenia is a deficiency of the number of white blood cells. The most common causes of leukopenia are: impairment of white blood cell production by environmental poisons, chemotherapeutic drugs, radiation therapy, and some hereditary diseases. Low white blood cell count can be reversed with astragalus. In fact, this is one of the most common uses of astragalus in the clinical practice of doctors of traditional Chinese medicine (TCM). Reversing both red and white blood cell deficiencies caused by modern medical treatments that have anemia or leukopenia as a side effect is a routine part of TCM practice.[8]

In clinical practice, astragalus is often combined with Angelica sinensis, known commonly by its Mandarin name dang gui (tang kwei). This combination, known as dang gui bue xin tang, has been studied in over a dozen scientific investigations.[9,10] In each study the combination of the two herbs worked better than either one alone to reverse anemia and leukopenia. Several studies have looked at what would be the best ratio of astragalus to dang gui in the formula. It has been determined that the best ratio of the two herbs together is five parts astragalus to one part dang gui for anemia, leukopenia, and the building of blood vessels.[11-13] Research has revealed why astragalus and dang gui have synergy together. A chemical in dang gui, called ferrulic acid, increases the permeability of cell membranes to astragalus. What that means is that dang gui opens up the membranes of cells specifically to allow isoflavonoids of astragalus to enter cells easier and be much stronger in their effects. This puts dang gui in the scientific category called a "doorman drug". That is it opens up a door, here being cellular membranes, to allow better absorption into cells. Ferrulic acid also helps make astragalus more soluble. This increases absorption of astragalus as well. It is interesting to note that the 5:1 ratio in these studies was the exact amount recommended 1,000 years ago by doctors of traditional Chinese medicine. It is also vital that the dang gui be cooked, optimally in wine. This type of cooking alters the molecular structure of this herb and activates it.[14,15]

Several other astragalus-based herbal combinations designed to reverse anemia and leukopenia have been researched as well. In 2007 researchers looked to see if the traditional Chinese medicine Huang Qi Liu Yi Tang could reverse the immunosuppression caused by the drug cyclophosphamide (Cytoxin). This combination of astragalus, licorice, and jujube dates significantly reversed immune suppression and dramatically increased white blood cell levels to normal.[16] In another important study it was shown that combining astragalus with Panax notoginseng (tian qi) produces impressive bone marrow stem cell production and EPO generation.[17] There are little or no side effects with any of these herbal combinations.

Several years ago a young girl, "Ann" 12 years old, was brought into my office by her parents with a very serious health problem. She had received tuberculosis chemotherapy that had severely damaged her bone marrow causing aplastic anemia. Some medications can damage bone marrow and prevent the production of both red and white blood cells. With aplastic anemia blood production is significantly shut down and can be fatal. Ann looked and acted ill, with a waxy pallor and severe fatigue. Ann's parents were at their wits ends. After seeing me they were scheduled to see their family physician to discuss the possibility of a bone marrow transplant. I had just seen a patient who owned an elk antler ranch in Montana. He told me that Korean scientists had recently harvested antlers from elk on his ranch. He generously gave me several bottles of elk antler extract. Antlers, unlike horns, fall off and regenerate every year. This takes a monumental ability to grow antler tissue very rapidly. Chemicals deposited inside the antlers are a source of blood cell generating nutrients. I had utilized antler extract several times in the last few years, mostly for osteoporosis and fracture healing. Over several years I had read a few studies of antler extract improving anemias and decided that this was an opportunity to help this girl with her life threatening anemia. I prescribed astragalus combined with the antler extract. I vividly remember receiving a phone call from the father the next day telling me that their physician reprimanded them for trying what he thought was a silly idea, and that this natural combination of astragalus and antler extract would do nothing for their daughter. The parents and physician finally came to an agreement that while the physician would begin the task of moving forward with finding a match for Ann's bone marrow, she could take the astragalus-antler combination. In a very dramatic occurrence, the antler-astragalus combination immediately began to stimulate Ann's bone marrow, increasing the production of red blood cells. In one month her red blood cell count rose to near normal. Two month later she was completely recovered, much to the delight of her parents and surprise of her physician.

Chapter 5

CANCER

Cancer is the number two cause of death in the United States. The vast majority of cancers (about 90%) are environmentally caused. This means that toxic chemicals in our diet and environment are mutating cells, turning on cancer genes, and creating solid tumors as well as blood cancers such as lymphoma and leukemia. For example, if one considers that for the last 70 years we have been spraying our food with some of the most poisonous chemicals ever developed it is not surprising to see this rise in cancer. The DDT family of insecticides called organochlorides, were developed in the mid 20th century. They persist in the environment for a very long time. Scientists from the Environmental Protection Agency have sampled soil from farms that have not used DDT or its sister chemicals for several decades. What the scientists discovered was that even after the chemicals were banned, they still remained intact in the soil ready to be taken up by plants and eaten by us. Organochlorides are still accumulating in the ocean environment as well, especially in farmed fish. It is becoming more and more difficult to avoid this family of pesticides. Atlantic farmed salmon, for example, contains 2 to 11 times the amount of these persistent pesticides as wild salmon.[1]

Because of their fat loving chlorine-based chemistry, organochloride chemicals are stored in our body's fat cells for months or even years. During periods of fasting or dieting they are partially released from our fat cells. They circulate around our bodies creating havoc, and then are mostly reabsorbed and stored in fat cells again, only to be released to circulate over and over again in the future. We have little ability to break down these pesticides, and they remain intact and potentially carcinogenic to us for a very long time.[2] They can also significantly damage immune and neurological function.[3] There is a strong link between organochloride pesticides and breast cancer.[4] Studies show that almost every person in the United States has traces of organochlorides in their bodies. Because of their toxicity and persistence in the environment and our bodies, almost all of the manufacturing of organochloride pesticides has now been banned in the United States. Other countries, however, do still manufacture them and we can end up ingesting them in some imported foods. David Weir and Marc Shapiro's landmark book *Circle of Poison* documents this phenomenon.[5]

The next generation of carcinogenic pesticides developed are in the chemical family called organophosphates. These phosphorus containing chemicals were originally developed by German scientists in the late 1930's in an attempt to produce stronger pesticides. Most of these pesticides, including the now infamous Sarin, were found too toxic for people to even touch or breath. So attention was turned to researching Sarin and other organophosphates to be utilized in World War II as a possible new and improved substitute for cyanide in warfare. Another goal was to find more efficient ways to murder death camp inmates during the holocaust. We are now, and have been for more than half a century, eating food containing Nazi nerve gas chemicals.[6]

Organophosphates were introduced to farmers to take the place of the DDT family of pesticides because they do not accumulate over a long time. But they do exist in foods for several weeks to months. Studies show that these phosphate insecticides remain intact long enough to be absorbed by people eating foods sprayed with them. Their contamination in food and absorption by people have been reported in almost every scientific study that has looked for this. There is evidence that astragalus can be helpful in reducing organophosphate toxicity. Studies show that astragalus significantly reduces the respiratory distress and heart and nervous system dysfunction that occur from organophosphate pesticide exposure.[7] This is particularly important because, although organophosphate pesticides do not accumulate in the environment as long as the organochloride pesticides, they are generally more toxic. By substituting organophosphates for organochlorides in the 1970's we traded moderately toxic long lasting pesticides for highly toxic short lived ones.[8]

Organochloride and organophosphate pesticides both kill pests by inhibiting acetylcholinesterase, which is the enzyme we produce to counteract the neurotransmitter acetylcholine. Acetylcholine causes muscles to contract and the esterase allows for these contractions to be controlled by relaxing muscles. These pesticides interfere with the esterase enzyme. Pest's nervous systems are literally fried by the unimpeded electrical impulses that build up in their nervous system causing constant uncontrolled spasming and seizuring. A summary of my doctoral thesis, *Treatment of Pesticide Poisoning with Acupuncture*, appearing in the December 1985 edition of the *American Journal of Acupuncture*, discusses these two insecticide groups in detail.[9]

Besides pesticides and other petroleum industry created chemicals, the most common cancer risk is from cigarettes. Cigarettes contain hundreds of toxic chemicals, including the rarely mentioned radioactive nuclide polonium. Yes, cigarettes are highly radioactive. Polonium is a breakdown product from high potassium fertilizers, and has an affinity for tobacco leaves. Polonium is an alpha emitter. That is, polonium emits or "spits" a particular kind of radiation called alpha particles. Alpha emitters are the most toxic substances on the face of the earth. They are 2,500,000% more toxic than hydrogen cyanide. When alpha particles are inhaled, they potentially damage, mutate, and kill normal lung cells or any other live cell they come in contact with. Think of fireworks going off in your lungs, except with alpha particles the fireworks are nuclear missiles.

In an important study conducted by the UCLA School of Medicine in 2012, researchers utilized secret information that cigarette companies were forced to reveal by a court settlement agreement. In this study it was shown that cigarette company executives knew about the dangers of radioactive polonium in cigarettes in the 1950's. They hid the fact that a simple acid wash of tobacco leaves could remove most of the polonium before it reached consumers. Since that acid wash was also found to reduce the speed in which nicotine was absorbed, cigarette company executives decided to not utilize the decontaminating acid wash. They did this because they were afraid that smokers would not get a quick enough nicotine high. The UCLA researchers found that the polonium alone in cigarettes causes 128-135 cancer deaths per 1000 smokers per year.[10] That is about one and a half million lung cancer deaths per year worldwide just from the polonium. Cigarette company executives continually hid the information that showed that they were aware that cigarettes could be made less deadly. It is a disgrace is that no one has ever been prosecuted for knowingly increasing the risk of death to millions of people.

Another common alpha emitter is radon, which seeps from granite kitchen counter tops, concrete basement walls, and foundations. Next are the myriad of synthetic chemicals developed in the last 50 years that cause cancer. Many toxic synthetic chemicals signal our cells to turn cancerous. It is important to note that the body usually does what it's told. When you smoke a cigarette, you are in fact ordering up cancer. It is up to your body's immune system to cancel that order.

So how can we protect ourselves from environmental cancer causing chemicals? First, reduce as much as possible the exposure to them. Eating food that is organically grown is a good start. There are many studies that show that organically raised food is higher in nutrition and tastes better than pesticide laden food.[11,12] There is a very big push back from food companies on these studies. They continue to state that conventionally grown produce is just as safe and healthy as organically raised food. Scientific committees, often paid by food and chemical companies, put out statements claiming that there is no proof that organically raised food is better than conventionally raised food. To get to these opinions these groups merely ignore or throw out any studies that disagree with the corporate view. To complicate this issue, some teachers at agriculture based colleges and universities also try to persuade consumers that the difference between organic food and conventionally raised food is insignificant. Having been an agriculture student in college myself, I see a formidable link between agriculture colleges and the chemical companies that often help fund them. It is true that because the world is so polluted now, the difference between organic and conventionally raised foods is becoming smaller. It is getting harder and harder to grow food that has only traces of toxic pesticides. All the more reason to protect ourselves with nutrients such as astragalus that reduce the risk of cancer and other diseases from synthetic pesticides.

Children are very susceptible to pollution damage largely due to their high metabolic rates and incompletely developed immune systems. Studies show that children rapidly absorb pesticides from foods and their blood levels of these toxic compounds go up when eating conventionally raised food and go down dramatically when organic food is consumed.[13] This is especially concerning as children's brains and immune systems are developing rapidly. It seems reasonable that the chronic ingestion of immunotoxic and neurotoxic chemicals should be reduced as much as possible in this age group. In my view, the significant increase in childhood cancer, autism, and hyperactivity that has occurred in the last thirty years could be caused in part by continually consuming food with traces of carcinogenic and neurotoxic pesticides.

Besides reducing toxin exposure, another way to protect us from cancer-causing chemicals is to utilize nutrients that are antioxidant and anti-tumorogenic. Antioxidant chemicals protect us from pollution by preventing electrons from being ripped away from atoms in our cells. Picture our solar system with its central sun and orbiting planets. Atoms are the same idea, a central nucleus and orbiting electrons. Many synthetic chemicals steal electrons away from atoms that make up our cells, which can either kill the cells, mutate them, or disrupt their function. Antioxidant foods and supplements protect our cells from this stealing of our electrons. Hundreds of antioxidant chemicals in foods have already been discovered. Fruits and vegetables that are colored purple, blue, red, orange, and yellow contain substances called flavonoids. They are antioxidant and healing. One antioxidant rich food is astragalus. The flavonoids in astragalus are one way in which we can receive this health building effect. Besides flavonoids, the saponin chemicals in astragalus, especially astragaloside IV, have been shown to reduce cancer occurrence in scientific studies and help slow cancer growth if it does occur. The starches in astragalus, called polysaccharides, are vital as well, dramatically increasing immune function. It is important to note that while isoflavonoids are the most antioxidant of astragalus' components, its saponins and polysaccharides are also antioxidants.

Astragalus also has a remarkable effect of often making both chemotherapeutic drugs and radiation therapy work better and with less side effects in the treatment of cancer.[14] In an example of this, researchers at Guangxi Medical University in Nanning China wanted to see if a combination of astragalus with ginseng could enhance the effectiveness of the common chemotherapeutic drug 5-FU (flourourcil). In the experiment, researchers found that the combination of astragalus and ginseng significantly increased the ability of the chemotherapeutic drug 5-FU to cause gastric cancer cells to stop proliferating, and instead to turn off and die. 5-FU is utilized in very serous cancers such as pancreatic, inflammatory breast, and colon. Adding this astragalus combination to this common chemotherapeutic 5-FU compound could dramatically increase the effectiveness of treatment.[15]

Astragalus is a food that can give a patient a better quality of life during cancer treatment. Astragalus reduces cancer treatment's destruction of bone marrow and red and white blood cells. Some cancer physicians are concerned that adding any nutrient that is antioxidant will reduce radiation therapy's ability to kill cancer cells. The opposite is true with astragalus. It does not protect cancer cells from radiation and actually enhances its toxic effect on tumors and leukemia, while protecting normal cells from radiation poisoning.[16] Again astragalus alters the body to be healthier at the appropriate time and place.

The liver filters chemicals from the bloodstream. Continually filtering environmental toxins often causes primary tumors to form in the liver. The liver is also an organ system that catches cancer cells floating through the bloodstream from cancerous organs. Astragalus has direct effects on reducing liver cancer caused by environmental toxins.[17] In a study by the International Agency for Research on Cancer in France, astragalus was found to both delay and reduce the induction of liver cancer.[18] Considering that liver cancer is over 90% fatal, there is a great need for prevention.

In an important study by the Clinical Pharmacy and Pharmacology Research Institute in Hunan, China, researchers report that astragalus polysaccharides, which are found in high concentrations in the roots, greatly enhance the ability of several commonly utilized chemotherapeutic drugs to kill liver cancer cells. They include cyclophosphamide, adriamycin, 5-flourouracil, cisplatin, etoposide, and vincristine. The researchers showed that Astragalus could turn off multidrug-resistant pumps (MDRs) in cancer cells. Cancer cells have actual pumps (efflux pumps) that pump out cancer medications as they are penetrating the cancer cells. Stopping the MDRs allows for the chemotherapeutic chemicals to enter cancer cells more easily and kill them much more effectively. In the study, increasing the dose of astragalus enhanced the anti-tumor effect of these cancer drugs dramatically.[19] Other studies have found the same cancer multidrug-resistance busting effect by astragalus.[20]

As mentioned, many oncologists are concerned that adding herbs such as astragalus to cancer treatment will reduce the efficacy of chemotherapy. One of the above studied drugs, adriamycin, works partially by enhancing oxidation to tumor cells. It is extremely useful against several classes of cancer including breast, lung, ovarian and blood cancers (lymphoma and leukemia). Unfortunately, it also kills heart cells very efficiently. In the most sophisticated investigation so far of astragalus' effect on adriamycin's cardiotoxicity, cancer researchers showed that astragaloside IV significantly protected heart cells by several different mechanisms. There was absolutely no interference with adriamycin's anti tumor actions.[21] This flies in the face of those who claim that herbs reduce the efficacy of chemotherapeutic drugs that rely heavily on oxidative stress as a weapon against cancer. If astragalus did interfere with chemotherapy oxidation, increasing the dose of astragalus would reduce treatment effectiveness. In the real world, it does the opposite.

A recent study in *Science Translational Medicine* in 2014 that received large amounts of publicity found that some antioxidants may interfere with the production of the protein p53 (cellular tumor antigen p53), which the body uses to turn off cancer cells through apoptosis, as well as repair damaged DNA. Astragalus has been shown to do the opposite. It up regulates the production of p53, increasing this important cancer fighting chemical.[22] Actually the most important aspect of p53 and human health is in ensuring it does not mutate through environmental damage from toxic chemicals, radiation, and viruses. Over half of all human tumors have mutated p53 in them. Astragalus is strongly anti-mutagenic and anti-viral and may offer some assistance to p53's stability.

MDRs are also mechanisms that are involved in antibiotic resistance. In antibiotic resistance, it's the bacteria, such as *Staph. aureus*, that have the multidrug-resistance pumps. These pumps within the bacteria push out the antibiotics. MRSA (Methylcillin Resistant *Staph. Aureus*) bacteria have very efficient pumps. That is one of the reasons they are so resistant to antibiotic therapy. MRSA also has a gene (mecA) that stops the breakdown of bacterial cell walls. Several herbs have been shown to turn off bacterial MDRs. Adding them to antibiotic therapy increases the effectiveness of that class of drugs. Unfortunately, no U.S. hospitals utilize this non-toxic approach to antibiotic resistant bacterial infections.

Astragalus fights cancer through several molecular mechanisms. It stimulates several immune system actions, including the significant enhancement of white blood cell's ability to recognize, move towards, and kill cancer cells. Imagine cancer genes trying to attach to normal cells to transform these normal cells into cancer cells. Astragalus interferes with the adherence of cancer genes on normal cells thus reducing cancer cells from getting a foothold on normal tissue. Astragalus also causes significant apoptosis of cancer cells.[23] Apoptosis is the switching off of cells. This is a process that occurs with normal cells (called programmed cell death) as a way of promoting new healthy cells to replace old weak cells.

In current cancer therapy, radiation and many chemotherapeutic drugs work only partly by apoptosis. Often, their main action is by what is called necrosis, the damaging and subsequent rotting of cells by a toxic chemical. Necrosis unfortunately also damages adjacent normal cells and causes significant inflammation. Radiation at high doses is very efficient at necrosis. Cancer therapies that rely on necrosis are some of the most toxic approaches as they kill many normal cells as collateral damage, and can mutate these normal cells to possibly turn cancerous in the near or distant future. Apoptosis causes no collateral damage, does not increase the risk of future therapy-caused cancers, and only turns off specific cells, here being cancer cells.

The irony of modern cancer therapy is that almost all chemotherapeutic drugs are strong carcinogens themselves and radiation treatment is actually one of the most potent cancer causing therapies in the world. It is a well known fact that modern cancer therapy has a significant risk of causing cancer several years after the therapy is over. In chemotherapy, the risk is greatest for the development of leukemias. It is important to reduce this possibility with an anti-cancer nutrient such as astragalus. Someday many cancer therapies will be apoptotic in nature, and necrotic treatment will be considered barbaric. Fortunately, many newer radiation techniques, especially concentrating gamma beams precisely at tumors, have begun to yield better and less toxic results. Astragalus has been shown to reverse the expression of the majority of genes mutated by irradiation.

Astragalus will probably not completely cure cancer in many people all by itself. But it does generally slow the rate of cancer growth and enhances other therapies to work better and with less side effects. In two examples of this, researchers working separately at the Loma Linda University School of Medicine in California and the University of Texas System Cancer Center looked to see if astragalus could increase the immune therapy action of interleukin-

2(IL-2), a synthetic immune enhancing chemical. As good as IL-2 is at activating killer cells to attack cancer, it is also very toxic, which limits its clinical value. Researchers wanted to see if, by adding astragalus to much smaller doses of IL-2, they could get better results with less side effects. What both research groups found was highly significant. Both groups found that astragalus increased the cancer killing potential of IL-2 by over 1000%.[24,25] **See chart**.

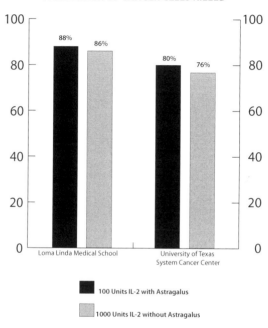

PERCENTAGE OF CANCER CELLS KILLED

The School of Pharmacy at the University of Mississippi recently tested to see if astragalus alone could enhance the natural production of IL-2 in mice. They reported that astragalus saponins could "create powerful immunoregulatory effects without the stimulation of inflammatory cytokines".[26] In one more study of IL-2, researchers at The Huasjan Hopsital in Shanghai measured astragalus side by side with IL-2 against lung cancer to see if immune cells called dendritic cells could be enhanced in their action of reducing the metastasis of lung cancer. What they found was that astragalus alone could slow the development of lung cancer just as well as IL-2.[27] Several other studies also find that adding astragalus to cancer treatment enhances chemotherapy and radiation therapy while reducing their toxic effects.

Even in terminally ill cancer patients astragalus has been shown to dramatically increase quality of life, allowing the cancer patient to experience less pain, better sleep, better appetite, longer lifespan, less fatigue, and more energy.[28] In a 2012 study researchers in China gave astragalus to cancer patients who had moderate to severe fatigue. In this very rigorous study (double-blind, randomized, placebo-controlled, crossover) almost all patients had a significant reduction in fatigue when using astragalus.[29]

Lack of appetite (anorexia) is a serious problem for people with cancer. Korean researchers investigated whether astragalus could help reverse anorexia in patients with advanced cancer. They found that by adding astragalus to the patients diet, appetite significantly improved.[30] It cannot be overemphasized how important it is for patients going through cancer therapy to feel as good as they possibly can. This actually helps therapies work better, partly by reducing cortisol that is created when we are stressed out and consumed by the negative feelings cancer and its challenging therapies produce. Immune function is generally much more efficient in a happy person than a depressed one. In those people who have incurable malignancy, astragalus offers the opportunity of exiting this world with reduced pain and discomfort.

In an interesting study from China, children with acute leukemia in remission were either given chemotherapy by itself or astragalus and chemotherapy combined. The scientists hoped that the astragalus would enhance dendritic cells to signal other immune cells to recognize and attack cancer cells. Dendritic cells are unique in that they send out long thin projections that extend between non-immune cells, almost like an immune system spider web.

Dendritic cells act as guardians of the body, often being the first line of attack when a foreign substance, such as cancer, is detected. Dendritic cells produce large amounts of a chemical called interleukin-12 (IL-12). High IL-12 levels shift the immune system to attack cancer cells. This is vitally important. Cancer cells have a trick up their sleeve in that they can slow down this IL-12 production which then allows the cancer cells to grow faster. As soon as a dendritic cell recognizes cancer it swiftly moves to a nearby lymph node and begins to produce the chemicals that help immune cells grow and directly fight the cancer. The better dendritic cells work, the better the immune system's early response to cancer. The children in the leukemia study who received astragalus showed a significant increase (almost doubling) of this dendritic immune function.[31]

DENDRITIC CELL

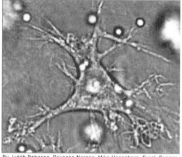

By Judith Behnsen, Priyanka Narang, Mike Hasenberg, Frank Gunzer, Ursula Bilitewski, Nina Klippel, Manfred Rohde, Matthias Brock, Axel A. Brakhage, Matthias Gunzer

In other studies on these dendritic cells, researchers also found out that astragalus increases the long protrusions of dendritic cells, making them much more active.[32] Another study found that astragalus induces dendritic cells to mature at an incredibly fast rate and be more sensitive and powerful in increasing immune function.[33] Astragalus not only effects dendritic cells ability to assist in conventional leukemia treatment but has a direct effect as well. Utilizing the flavonoids of astragalus, researchers have found that leukemia cell production is inhibited significantly even without additional immune support.[34] In another important study with astragalus and leukemia, researchers at the First Affiliated Hospital in Beijing found that the flavonoids of astragalus significantly inhibit human erythroleukemia proliferation.[35] This is a very important finding because this type of leukemia is usually fatal within three years of diagnosis.

In one of the most interesting studies on astragalus and dendritic cells, researchers looked to see if astragalus could alter either Lactobacillus acidophilus or E. coli's effect on immune response. Acidophilus and E. coli bacterias are both found in the intestinal tract. Some strains of E. coli in are not harmful in small numbers. But in large numbers they can give us life threatening inflammation and infections. In the Beijing Hospital experiment researchers found that E. coli increased inflammatory cytokines and astragalus treatment reduced that inflammatory response. Combining astragalus with acidophilus lead to an immune enhancing effect on dendritic cells by increasing interferon production dramatically. This is one of the first studies to show that astragalus and probiotics act powerfully together to increase immune function and anticancer and antiviral activity.[36]

NF KAPPA-B
(Nuclear factor-Kappa-light-chain-enhancer of activated B cells)

NF Kappa-B is a specialized protein that grabs specific sequences of DNA and changes them around. This creates activation and/or repression of many genes. Cells respond to those signals and are told what to do. In cancer NF Kappa B becomes deranged by gene mutations and increases tumor growth. Cancer cells also secrete factors that cause NF Kappa B to increase and this helps tumors to grow even more rapidly. Astragalus turns off deranged NF Kappa B and reduces the mutations that caused NF Kappa B to alter its function.

One way astragalus slows cancers growth is by suppressing a chemical compound known as NF-kappaB.[37] **See box.** NF-kappaB is secreted by cancer cells to help them thrive and shield themselves from anti-inflammatory and anticancer chemicals in the body. NF-kappaB also enhances cancer growth by promoting blood vessels to grow around the tumor site and in effect feed the tumor. This is called angiogenesis. Astragalus significantly turns off NF-kappaB in tumor cells and has been shown in several studies to starve cancer cells by reducing angiogenesis. This reduces the invasiveness of metastatic cancers. In fact, formononetin, a flavonoid of astragalus has been shown to completely eliminate the invasiveness of metastatic colon cancer.[38] Other chemicals that are involved in cancer angiogenesis are growth factor, MMP, and MMT. These are all reduced in the cancer cell environment by astragalus as well.[39]

It is important to note that this is the opposite of what happens in an injury when astragalus enhances blood vessel production to repair the damaged area. Once the area is healed, astragalus turns off angiogenesis to that area. Again astragalus alters the body towards health and away from disease. The ability for Astragalus to enhance several different immune functions, including increasing white blood cells recognition and attack of cancer cells, may be unmatched by any other medicine.[40-47]

Cancer cells can poison adjacent normal cells and astragalus inhibits this kind of destruction as well.[48] Tumors also produce other factors that suppress immune function. In a study done at the Department of Urology at Loma Linda University School of Medicine, researchers studied if astragalus could reverse this immune suppression in both bladder tumors and renal carcinoma. Without the addition of astragalus, macrophages (an important immune cell) did not attack cancer cells with much efficiency. But when astragalus was added to both bladder and kidney tumors, suppression of this immune function was reduced with a low astragalus dose and completely eliminated with a high dose.[49]

In an experiment to check on the molecular mechanisms involved with this tumor induced immune suppression, researchers at the Cancer Hospital of Tinjin Medical University in China looked at the genetic expression of Treg cells which are recruited into the tumor microenvironment. Treg cells (T regulator cells) suppress other immune cells. This can be helpful to reduce autoimmune diseases. But they can also suppress immune attack of cancer cells. What the cancer researchers found was that the polysaccharides in astragalus restore the balance of cytokines, the chemicals that help Treg cells suppress immune function. In the 31 patients with liver cancer, these Treg cells were present in all of them. Treg cells spit chemicals that help cancer grow by lowering immune response. The researchers found that astragalus changed the microenvironment of the tumor by blocking Treg cells from migrating into liver cancer tissue. By blocking these immune suppressing Treg cells, other immune cells can attack tumors much more powerfully.[50]

One astragalus containing supplement, called BreastDefend, is being touted by some physicians as an effective adjunctive therapeutic agent against invasive breast cancer. The latest study, by the Indiana University Cancer Research Laboratory, showed that BreastDefend reduced the size of triple-negative tumors in mice. Triple negative tumors are those that have no genes for estrogen receptor, progesterone receptor, or Her2/neu cancers. Some of these types of cancers can be very aggressive. Besides the challenge of getting the cancers to go into remission, the biggest obstacle in these cancers may be in preventing cancer relapse. In triple-negative cancers the risk for cancer relapse is very high in the first five years after cancer therapy. BreastDefend also decreased the incidence of breast to lung cancer metastasis from 67% in controls to 20% in the BreastDefend group. It also reduced the expression of two breast cancer genes. In another study with BreastDefend researchers report that metastatic breast cancer cells were significantly reduced in numbers.[51,52] It is difficult to know how much astragalus has to do with these impressive results. It is only one of 8 herbs and other nutrients in BreastDefend. Astragalus is about 12% of the formula. The recommended dose for active support is equivalent to about 2,000 mg. of astragalus root per day. This is well within the effective dosage range found in many cancer studies. Since triple negative cancers reappear at an alarming rate, BreastDefend may be quite helpful in reducing recurrence.

Some of the most interesting research now with cancer is to

find the genes that mutate and create specific cancers. Specific drugs can then be utilized for these specific mutations. The HER2 gene is an excellent example of a gene that can be targeted. It is responsible for about 20% of breast cancer. Chemotherapeutic medications have been developed (lapatinib and trastuzumab) that block this cancer producing gene. Other genes such as KRAS, that when mutated cause several different cancers, are being researched as well. This kind of research will help reduce the trial and error chemotherapeutic regimes that are now utilized in most cancer treatments. Research in this area is slow, mainly because research money is not flowing in from the pharmaceutical companies. This is because specific chemotherapeutic drugs and their diagnostic tests will not make drug companies as much money as the present day approach of guessing if a cancer drug will work and giving that drug to a vast amount of people. Targeted diagnostics and drugs will have specific markets that will be smaller than the market for a commonly used cancer drug like cisplatin is used right now. Instead of a huge amount of people utilizing the same cancer drug, small groups of cancer patients will be treated with one or more of dozens of individual targeting drugs. Pharmaceutical companies will have to develop more drugs and compete with other companies for a smaller market for that drug. The one caveat with this research is that cancer genes have already begun to show acquired resistance to some of these targeting anti-mutation drugs. New drugs will need to be created as resistance occurs. Astragalus may be of benefit to these specific treatments as it may amplify their anticancer effects and reduce side effects. Astragalus is a strong anti-mutagen, and has be shown to stop many different types of mutations that cause cancer.

As I write this chapter, I am thinking of a wonderful patient who has just died of metastatic breast cancer. Her physicians demanded that she not take any nutritional supplements, which also included denying my recommendation that she be allowed to take astragalus along with her chemotherapy and radiation treatments. She was taken care of at a well regarded breast health center at UC San Francisco. I am left to wonder if allowing her to augment her therapy with astragalus would have helped her. Her chemotherapeutic drugs are among those studied in astragalus research. Studies that show that astragalus could have increased the effectiveness of her therapy. How many people have to die before modern cancer centers begin to take advantage of astragalus and other herbs that could possibly make a difference for people struggling with this disease?

Astragalus has been shown in several studies to prevent and slow the growth of both solid tumors and blood cancers. It reduces chemotherapeutic and radiation therapies toxicities and often increases their effectiveness. Astragalus increases quality of life in all cancer patients, reducing pain, nausea, insomnia, anxiety, and depression. Disallowing cancer patients astragalus has no scientific basis. Oncologists that refuse to believe scientific research in this area are doing their patients a tremendous disservice. Hopefully, further interest in astragalus will inspire cancer physicians to utilize this important herbal medicine in the future. There is some room for optimism in this area. Recently, the Society of Integrative Oncology has undertaken the challenge of providing basic information to physicians on natural supplements, including astragalus, that many cancer patients are already utilizing on their own.[53]

Chapter 6

HEART DISEASE

Heart disease, specifically (hardening and narrowing of the coronary arteries) is the number one killer in the United States. Coupled with viral infection (myocarditis), hypertension, and congestive heart failure, among other heart problems, heart disease will eventually affect most Americans in their later years. Astragalus has a premier place in heart health management as it significantly protects the heart muscle and its arteries.[1-3] In atherosclerosis studies, astragalus directly dilates coronary arteries allowing more oxygen to the heart muscle.[4-6] This reduces the risk of a heart attack, as well as protecting cardiac tissue if a heart attack does occur.

In a study of heart attack victims by the University of Beijing Hospital, 43 patients who presented at the hospital were given astragalus within 36 hours of being admitted. Patients who received astragalus had significantly improved heart function and reduced heart damage. The free radical damage to the heart muscle was shown to be much lower than would be normally expected. The study showed that astragalus increased the patients production of the powerful antioxidant superoxide dismutase and improved left ventricular heart function.[7] A study at the Chinese Cardiovascular Research Institute found that astragalus is an effective anti-inflammatory agent that decreases the response by the immune system to attack and damage the lining of the arteries (endothelium). In the Cardiovascular Research Institute study astragalus significantly suppressed the progression of atherosclerosis.[8]

Possibly the most comprehensive study looking at all the different ways that astragalus helps reduce damage to heart tissue after a heart attack was performed at the State Key Laboratory of Natural and Biomemetic Drugs at Peking University in 2013. Researchers found that astragalus extract reduced the size and severity of damage to heart tissue and significantly decreased the release of cardiac enzymes that signal heart muscle damage. Heart function improved dramatically, with astragalus protecting tissue from loss of oxygen. As mentioned above, strong antioxidant chemicals are created from astragalus and it blocked heart cell death by stopping migration of excess calcium into the heart and more importantly by opening mitochondrial potassium channels into the heart which reduces cardiac tissue spasming and heart cell death. Mitochondria are the energy producing engines of the heart cells and it is vital that they remain at high function. By protecting the cardiac mitochondria, energy to the heart muscle is dramatically increased.[9]

In another hospital study in China, 92 patients with advanced coronary heart disease reported significant reduction in angina pain after receiving astragalus, and electrocardiogram (EKG) studies showed an average 82.6% improvement.[10] The EKG study is especially important as it is an objective finding that shows that astragalus is a powerful heart medicine even in advanced heart disease. When a heart attack occurs there is a huge amount of toxic chemicals produced at the site of coronary artery blockage. Heart tissue suddenly exists in an area with no oxygen or nutrient supply. When blood returns to this starved tissue, large amounts of oxygen and white blood cells flood into the formally oxygen deprived cells and cause an inflammatory response that is very damaging to tissue. White blood cells begin to spit free radical and other toxic chemicals causing heart cells to die. This is called reperfusion injury. Astragalus has been shown to protect the heart from reperfusion injury, greatly reducing heart damage.

Astragalus reduces blood pressure in those individuals with high blood pressure. This is not, as some authorities have stated, due to the mild diuretic action of astragalus. Studies done on astragalus show that even if large doses of astragalus are taken, and urination increases, there is no significant effect on blood pressure if it's in the normal range. It is also noteworthy to mention that astragalus spares potassium in its diuretic action.[11]

Astragalus also protects and heals heart tissue from damage from several viruses, especially coxsackie and adenovirus. These viruses cause severe inflammation and injury to heart cells. Astragalus reverses this. Called myocarditis or inflammatory cardiomyopathy, this heart disease is one of the most thoroughly studied astragalus interventions.[12-27]

As we age, our heart muscle can weaken due to coronary artery disease, high blood pressure, or viral attack. In a study by the department of cardiology at the Jinning Medical College Hospital in China, 84 patients with moderate to severe chronic heart failure were divided into two groups. Forty-two patients were given normal drug therapy and 42 patients were treated with astragalus. Although synthetic medication helped, the astragalus group improved significantly more than the drug group. Heart cells were preserved and protected by astragalus as seen by a decrease in heart cell death.[28] Several other studies have found astragalus prevents and reverses heart failure. In a study at Shanghai Medical University, nineteen patient with congestive heart failure received astragalus injections. After only two weeks of therapy, 75% of the patients reported complete remission of angina pain and labored breathing, and enjoyed a significant increase in exercise capacity. Detailed investigation revealed that astragalus improved both the structure and function of their hearts.[29] Many other studies have found similar results.[30-37]

Recent research with astragalus and myocardial hypertrophy showed that astragaloside IV strongly inhibited inflammatory cytokines leading to enhanced protection of heart tissue. Astragalus specifically inhibited NF-kappaB, as well as Toll-Like Receptor 4 (TLR4). These two proteins increase inflammatory immune responses that would damage heart cells. This is an excellent example where astragalus causes a protective shift away from a dangerous immune system attack on vital organ tissue.[38]

The most common cardiac intervention for people over 50 years old is reduction of cholesterol. Cholesterol is a vital compound that serves as a basic ingredient for the synthesis of Vitamin D, steroid hormones, bile acids, and cell membranes. Cholesterol is a type of waxy fat that is both consumed from animal products and synthesized mainly by the liver and circulates through our bloodstream. Our brains contain large amounts of cholesterol and fatty acids. You may be wondering if cholesterol is so important, why are physicians fighting so hard to reduce its concentration in our bloodstream. The reason is because cholesterol, under the right (wrong) conditions, has the potential to contribute to plaque buildup in our arteries and clog them up, causing a stroke or heart attack.

One issue that is seldom addressed is that cholesterol itself can become damaged through oxidation from environmental toxins, refined foods, and cigarettes. Eating foods high in sugar for example causes significant oxidation that turns cholesterol into a free radical generating compound that damages the inside of our blood vessels. Oxidized cholesterol is one of the most ignored aspects of heart disease. If people were healthier with more antioxidants in their diet, cholesterol would not be oxidized at nearly the rate it is now for most people.

Over the last twenty years drug companies have developed medications to reduce cholesterol levels. Statin drugs have now become the primary synthetic medications used to reduce cholesterol. They are among "The Holy Grail" of drugs for pharmaceutical companies as they are prescribed for life, giving the companies steady customers for many years. These drugs work by inhibiting a protein called HMG-CoA reductase. This chemical is responsible, in part, for creating cholesterol in the liver. By inhibiting this chemical we in turn make less cholesterol and blood levels go down. This inhibiting of HMG-CoA reductase, however, has a very dark side. This protein is also responsible for the creation of a chemical called Coenzyme Q10 or CoQ10. CoQ10 is one of the most important chemicals our bodies manufacture. It is responsible for creating energy deep within our cells in a compartment known as the mitochondria. Mitochondria are the energy creating engines of cells, making ATP (adenosine triphosphate) which fuels our metabolism. When a statin drug is taken, production of COQ10 goes down, because statins inhibit HMG-CoA reductase. The liver and muscles are often the first areas to show this energy starvation, and muscle fatigue and pain (which can become chronic even after discontinuing statins) are seen with about 10% of people taking statin drugs such as Lipitor. The question that is seldom asked is do statin drugs really lower the risk of heart attacks? A very important study that most people have never heard of is the JUPITER study. Published in 2010 in the *Archives of Internal Medicine* the study showed there was no difference in rate of heart attack incidence between people taking statin drugs and those receiving placebo.[39] The use of statins remains controversial. Several studies show conflicting data.

Scientists looking to see if the starches from astragalus could lower cholesterol levels without affecting the COQ10 pathway, gave a population of hamsters who had very high cholesterol levels a diet which included astragalus polysaccharides. The results were impressive. At the end of the three month trial, cholesterol and low density lipoprotein (LDL) levels dropped by almost one half. The HMG-CoA reductase pathway was not involved for this cholesterol reduction. No side effects were seen.[40]

Looking to see what molecular mechanisms might be responsible for astragalus lowering cholesterol and more importantly reducing cardiovascular disease, researchers at the PLA General Hospital in Beijing studied astragalus's effects in both laboratory animals and in test tube experiments. They found that the isoflavonoids of astragalus reduced total cholesterol and LDL cholesterol and increased beneficial HDL cholesterol. Even more important, astragalus was able to reduce the formation of what is called the fatty streak by up to 64%. The fatty streak is the initial damage to the inside of arteries. Toxic oxidative chemicals actually cut the inside of the arteries and begin a cascade of inflammation. White blood cells (mostly macrophages) follow oxidized cholesterol into the arteries and attempt to eat and remove it. The macrophages actually contribute significantly to oxidation of LDL cholesterol and make the inflammation much worse. Unfortunately the macrophages become overwhelmed with the job and swell up so much with oxidized cholesterol (specifically LDL) that they look like they are foaming at the mouth. They then become deranged and begin to hurt us instead of helping. Scientists call them foam cells. It's these foam cells that worsen fatty streaks. This includes the body trying to heal this damage by slapping cholesterol "bandages" on top of it. This piling on of fatty streaks eventually narrows arteries and can trap blood cells leaking from small ruptures in arteries as well as cholesterol chunks, causing a heart attack or stroke. In this study researchers showed that astragalus scavenged the oxidative chemicals that would normally begin this process of atherosclerosis. Astragalus shut down the atherosclerotic process.[41]

Another research group found that astragalus significantly reduces cardiovascular inflammation and those molecular mechanisms responsible for this could be measured. This study on mice showed that astragalus strongly inhibited the production of NF-kappaB and other chemicals responsible for early inflammation and progression of atherosclerosis.[42] Researchers at the Shanghai Institute of Cardiovascular Diseases found that a combination of astragalus, sage (*Salvia miltiorrhiza*), and dang gui (*Angelica sinensis*) was able to significantly reduce atherosclerosis and lower cholesterol and triglycerides in laboratory mice.[43] If these results could be duplicated in humans, an effective nontoxic astragalus-based cholesterol-lowering medication could be the outcome. In the meantime, taking whole root astragalus as a supplement could significantly reduce the injury and aging of arteries and heart muscle tissue.

Some researchers believe that we are lowering our cholesterol levels too much. There is mounting evidence that lowering cholesterol to very low levels increases the risk of a heart rhythm abnormality called atrial fibrillation (afib). Several studies have shown older adults who have low cholesterol levels have more problems with atrial fibrillation.[44,45] Other studies have found that low cholesterol levels are associated with early death.[46,47] The ENHANCE trial of 2008 utilized Vytorin as a cholesterol lowering statin medication. It worked very well to reduce cholesterol. In the trial, however, study participants had a highly significant increase in arterial plaque formation. So even though cholesterol levels diminished, an actual increase of atherosclerotic heart disease was seen.[48] The lesson being that focusing only on lowering cholesterol with statin drugs and not addressing diet, exercise, inflammation, and oxidation is short sighted and may actually worsen the risk for heart attacks, especially in those people over 50 years old. The truth is heart disease can be prevented in most people if they would exercise and eat a plant-based diet throughout their lives.

Chapter 7

THE BRAIN AND NERVOUS SYSTEM

Much of the research on astragalus and brain function has focused on the prevention and treatment of strokes (cerebral vascular accidents) and concussions. During and just after a stroke significant damage to brain cells can occur due to the cutting off of oxygen to this delicate tissue. Astragalus has been shown to reduce brain damage from strokes by increasing antioxidants in brain cells (neurons).[1] Strokes cause a huge production of free radical chemicals. Brain tissue is very susceptible to this kind of damage partly because of its high concentration of polyunsaturated fats, and polyunsaturated fats are very fragile. The brain has a defense of its own called the blood-brain barrier that screens chemicals and prohibits the incursion of toxic compounds into the brain. When a stroke occurs the blood-brain barrier is compromised, and toxic free radical chemicals that normally can't get into the brain can now sneak in and damage or kill brain cells. China has an Institute for Functional Brain Disorders. Scientists at the Institute studied astragalus's effects upon the blood-brain barrier after strokes. They found that astragalus protects the blood-brain barrier and significantly reduces the migration of toxic chemicals into the brain.[2]

Astragalus enhances the recovery of strokes, especially when combined with acupuncture. The National Institutes of Health state that acupuncture is of significant value in speeding the repair of brain tissue after strokes. I have found that the combination of acupuncture and astragalus can be incredibly effective in recovering from strokes. Although no scientific studies have been performed combining acupuncture with astragalus at present, there is good evidence that astragalus alone is of tremendous value in stroke rehabilitation. In a double blind, placebo controlled, randomized study testing the effects of astragalus on acute hemorrhagic stroke, 68 patients were followed for 12 weeks. One half of the group received 3 grams of astragalus per day and the other half of the group received a placebo. After twelve weeks the patients were assessed for mental and physical function. The patients in the astragalus group showed an almost doubling of mental and physical recovery compared to the placebo group.[3] Imagine the billions of dollars in healthcare savings alone that would occur if post-stroke patients were routinely given astragalus as a healing medicine.

Confusion, loss of memory, chronic depression, violent behavior, and serious neurological damage can occur after severe brain trauma from single or multiple concussions. Thirty years ago, physicians were taught that brain cells cannot regenerate once they were damaged. We now know that is not true. Now in the 21st century, through electron microscopy and sophisticated chemical analysis, we can see the genetic expression and molecular mechanisms at work when astragalus is utilized to regenerate neurons.[4] Neurites are projections (axons and dendrites) at the ends of nerve cells (neurons). They propel or accept electrical impulses along nerves. In experiments testing if astragalus could facilitate the regeneration of neurites after brain injuries, researchers have found that astragalus repairs neurites, and decreases memory disorders, effectively reversing brain damage.

Researchers at the Institute of Natural Medicine in Nantong, China wanted to see if astragalus combined with arctic root (*Rhodiola*) could be helpful in treating brain injuries similar to strokes and concussions. They found that the astragalus-rhodiola mixture prevented brain damage by inhibiting free radical and lactic acid chemicals from building up in the brain.[5] Scientists at Hubei Medical University in China also found that astragalus prevented the brain cells of rats from being damaged from lack of oxygen, called hypoxia.[6] This is extremely important because injuries to the brain from trauma such as concussion and strokes occur partly due to a cut off of oxygen to fragile brain cells. Often underrated is the damage that occurs when blood returns to the area. Additional injury results from abruptly high oxygen tension causing increased oxidation, temporary autoimmunity, and cellular damage. This is called reperfusion injury. It is the same type of injury previously described with heart attacks. Astragalus both prevents and significantly repairs reperfusion injury.

In the late 1980's a physician came into my office the day after having been hit by a car while he was riding his bicycle. He wasn't wearing a helmet (he admitted to being foolhardy). He had landed on the pavement head first and suffered a significant concussion. The left side of his face became completely paralyzed. After being taken to the local hospital emergency room for CAT scan and neurological evaluation, he refused to be admitted into the hospital and instead said he wanted to see if acupuncture and herbal medicine would help his injury. I gave him a large dose of astragalus right there and began to give him an acupuncture treatment for his trauma. In one of the most dramatic recoveries from a concussion I have ever seen, his face immediately began to regain muscle tone. In one hour his face was nearly recovered from the paralysis. He continued to take astragalus for one week and made a full recovery.

It would be interesting to give long term doses of astragalus to professional football players, boxers, rugby players, soccer players, etc. They receive hundreds of minor head traumas and many serious concussions throughout their careers. Preventing concussions and the brain damage that occurs with them should be a priority in these groups.

Alcoholism is a major problem in the United States. Millions of Americans consistently overconsume alcohol. Besides the stresses of modern society, genetic factors play a key role in many people's inability to stop drinking. After working in an alcohol and drug treatment center for three years giving over 8,000 acupuncture treatments there, I saw the damage first hand, not only to personal and work related relationships, but also the massive destruction that large amounts of alcohol does to the physical health of these individuals. Besides liver damage, alcohol also damages kidney and brain cells. Brain damage slowly develops and memory and cognitive functions suffer eventual decline. In a preliminary study looking to see if astragalus could reduce alcohol induced memory deficits, Chinese researchers found that astragalus was significantly effective in reducing alcohol related memory disorders.[7]

We normally break down alcohol in a two step process that renders it harmless. But when someone drinks too much at once or continually, alcohol byproducts called acetylaldehydes build up in the brain and cause toxicity.[8] This is caused specifically because the body is unable to break down alcohol fast enough, often due to a deficiency of acetylaldehyde dehydrogenase, one of the two enzymes responsible for alcohol detoxification.[9] The other enzyme is alcohol dehydrogenase. Both of these enzymes are zinc dependent. This means that if zinc is low in the diet, it won't be around to handle alcohol. Zinc is a common mineral deficiency for two reasons. First because it is not available in processed food. It is removed from grains when they are processed. And second, zinc is a part of about 50 proteins, called metalloenzymes, in the body. It is used up quickly for many important actions and is required regularly in the diet. In individuals who eat a processed food diet, chronic zinc deficiency is common. Acetylaldehydes are very toxic to brain cells. Acetylaldehydes are also the main reason for the hangover feeling when people drink too much. Dehydration is involved in the hangover feeling, but only because alcohol is not broken down into water fast enough to prevent toxicity. The phrase, "Take zinc when you drink", is true. Adding astragalus would increase protection of brain, kidney, and liver tissues.

Other toxic chemicals can damage brain tissue as well. Researchers in China found that astragalus protects brain and nerve tissue from damage by xanthines. These chemicals are the source of stimulants such as caffeine, and can cause heart arrhythmia and convulsions when delivered in large amounts. The isoflavonoids in astragalus were found to protect brain and nerve tissue significantly, with their main effects being inducing the body to make antioxidant chemicals such as superoxide dismutase (SOD) and glutathione peroxidase (GSH-Px).[10]

Deep in the brain of people developing Parkinson's Disease (PD), cells in an area called the substantia nigra are being attacked by oxidizing chemicals. Genetic susceptibility and toxins have combined to poison these brain cells. When the poisoning begins substantia nigra cells become damaged and cannot produce dopamine, a brain chemical that helps control movement. As the disease progresses people find they cannot move quickly anymore. They begin to shake when they are resting, their muscles become rigid, and it becomes difficult to walk, maintain balance, or even speak clearly. The disease slowly continues until many people find they cannot function without significant amounts of help. How does PD begin?

There is a lot of interesting research that points to toxins as being the trigger and/or accelerator for this disease. One of the possibilities is found in the intestinal tract. People with PD often have chronic low grade inflammation and a very leaky gut that is riddled with large amounts of the bacteria called E. Coli. E. Coli are normal residents of the intestinal tract when in low numbers. When they begin to take over as the king of the bacterial hill in the gut, problems begin. Nerve cells in the intestinal tract (the gut brain) show PD damage first from being directly poisoned by the toxins associated with overly large amounts of E. Coli.[11] This bacteria contains a poison called an endotoxin. Endotoxins are actually fat-sugar compounds in the outer membranes of E. Coli that help the bacteria to cling to our intestines. As these bacteria break down, their membrane skeletons poison us with endotoxins and create a huge immune response. This inflammatory response directly kills many of the 100 million neurons in the intestines. The brain cells are poisoned next. We have about 86 billion neurons in the brain. They are very fragile. It is important to note these particular bacteria love a high protein meat-based environment in our intestines. If an individual has a diet high in meat and low in fruits and vegetables they are basically farming toxic poisonous bacteria in very large numbers. This enables bacterial endotoxins to cause huge amounts of inflammation, cell death, and cancer. A chronically inflamed gastrointestinal tract also allows for large molecules of incompletely digested food particles to pass into the bloodstream. This can cause an additional immune response that is debilitating due to its length and subsequent disruption of normal physiology. Parkinson's Disease may be worsened or even partly caused by this type of bacterial imbalance. Several other toxins are also being studied. This inflammatory disease affects over 3 million Americans over the age of 65.

In a study done at Hong Kong Baptist University, researchers wondered if astragalus would be helpful in preventing or improving Parkinson's disease. In their study, they found massive brain cell death and degenerated brain cells in the substantia nigra. Using an isolated chemical from astragalus called astragaloside IV, scientists found that astragaloside IV protected neurons from damage and actually caused sprouting of new neurites, the ends of nerve cells.[12] Researchers at the Department of Neurosurgery in the Tangdu Hospital in China found that astragaloside IV could significantly protect brain cells and prevent the type of oxidative damage that occurs with Parkinson's disease.[13] These are exciting findings and show that astragalus may be useful for preventing and treating Parkinson's disease.

Another dreaded neurological illness is Alzheimer's Disease. It is now the 6th leading cause of death in the United States. In Alzheimer's disease, brain tissue is destroyed by toxic chemicals. Several chemicals are being studied, the principle one being a protein called amyloid. Amyloids are very toxic to brain tissue and significantly damage memory in Alzheimer's patients. At first researchers thought that amyloid plaque buildup in the brain was the offending agent. That led to a vaccine against the plaque. It worked well in lab animals, almost completely preventing amyloid plaque buildup. But unfortunately this had no helpful effect on memory and cognitive thinking. Another amyloid peptide that does not produce plaque buildup is more likely the toxin that, at least in part, causes Alzheimer's Disease. In a study with mice to see if astragalus could reduce brain damage from these amyloid peptides, Japanese researchers found astragalus induced brain cells to regenerate even after they were severely damaged by amyloid. Equally important, astragalus protected brain cells from early damage due to amyloid exposure. The mice in the study who received astragalus did not have the memory loss expected from amyloid poisoning, and instead had normal brain activity.[14]

One of the brain areas specifically damaged during the slow development of Alzheimer's disease is called the hippocampus. The hippocampus stores recent memories. It is one of the few areas of the brain that can regenerate neurons efficiently throughout our life. This is of vital importance as the hippocampus is extremely susceptible to damage by stress. In post-traumatic stress disorder for instance, it is the hippocampus that is damaged by the initial stresses of physical or mental abuse, warfare participation, or any other significant negative event or series of events. It then begins to cause mental changes such as depression and/or schizophrenia. These diseases then begin to damage the hippocampus themselves. Fortunately, astragalus can help reverse this hippocampus destruction. In a study to see if astragalus could protect this delicate tissue from the oxidative stress caused by lack of oxygen, astragalus had a strong protective effect on hippocampus tissue, dramatically reducing brain damage.[15] Two recent studies from Anhui Medical University in China show that astragalus protects brain tissue from stress hormones and from amyloid deposits. In these studies astragalus was able to prevent learning and memory impairments, reduce amyloid deposition in the hippocampus, and stop brain cells from dying.[16,17]

These interesting findings suggest that astragalus may be of help in preventing and treating this devastating disease. No single health factor stands out as being causative by itself. But people who are chronically ill with diabetes, heart disease, and poor health in general have a much greater chance of developing it. It appears that, at least in some people, Alzheimer's disease is accelerated due to the creation of a toxic environment within the body and brain specifically. Chronic exposure to aluminum, once considered a key toxin causing Alzheimer's disease, does cause severe neurological damage, and is responsible for a variant of Alzheimer's disease called ALS-PDC.[18]

A sedentary lifestyle and eating a processed food high sugar diet increases the risk for Alzheimer's Disease. Chronic disease enhances the disruption of normal brain function and may pave the way for abnormal amounts of amyloid. N-APP (amyloid precursor protein) and DR-6 (death receptor 6) are also created during Alzheimer's development. They cause brain cells to self destruct. Abnormal cell supporting proteins (Tau proteins), and other toxic compounds that destroy mental function are also involved with this disease. The ability of astragalus to protect brain tissue from toxins is very significant. It could be very valuable in Alzheimer's prevention and treatment.

Epilepsy is a poorly understood health problem. People who struggle with this disease often find that medications for epilepsy can be toxic and that side effects can often reduce their quality of life. Astragalus has a significant anti-seizure effect. At the Chinese Institute of Mitochondrial Biology and Medicine, researchers found that astragalus significantly reduces seizures by protecting against oxidative damage to the nervous system allowing for normal brain activity.[19] Researchers with the Mongolian Academy of Medicine attempted to see if Astragalus could be used to prevent seizures induced by the powerful epilepsy causing drug pentylenetetrazole. Astragalus was extraordinarily effective in preventing drug induced seizures in this study. This is, at least in part, due to astragalus protecting hippocampus brain cells as described in the Alzheimer's information section above. The hippocampus is the area of the brain that both causes and is injured by epileptic seizures. In the study, it was also noted that astragalus did not cause incoordination or sedation, common side effects seen with many synthetic anti-seizure medicines.[20] Many of my patients who have epilepsy find that taking astragalus either reduces or eliminates their need for anti-seizure medication. Reducing anti-seizure medication requires close monitoring of patients. An improvement in electroencephalograph (EEG) readings is the necessary objective finding allowing for the reduction or elimination of anti-seizure medication. In this way reduction or elimination of medication can take place slowly and safely.

Many people suffer injuries or diseases that cause damage to the nerves outside the brain and spinal cord. Called peripheral nerves, they have some modest ability to regenerate after being injured. That repair and regeneration is often very slow and can be complicated by chronic inflammation and subsequent scarring. Astragalus has been shown to be a nerve growth-promoting factor, speeding growth of both brain and peripheral nerve cells at a rate much faster than without astragalus.[21] Slow inefficient nerve repair often leads to lifelong pain and discomfort. Astragalus can improve nerve injuries due to trauma, diseases such as diabetes (peripheral neuropathy), and environmental damage such as exposure to certain herbicides and insecticides.

Chapter 8

LIVER

The liver is an amazing organ. It has many functions, including manufacturing hundreds of important chemicals and filtering toxins from our blood. This remarkable organ also has the potential to regenerate itself if given the right conditions. A human infant for example, has the capacity to regenerate almost all of its liver function if damaged. In laboratory experiments, young rodents who have most of their liver tissue removed are able to completely regenerate their liver function as well. We do lose some of the efficiency of liver repair as we get older, but we can still significantly regenerate damaged liver tissue as adults. This regeneration potential is important as we humans seem to regularly beat up, inflame, and kill our liver cells with all our toxic food, alcohol, drugs, and pollutants. Astragalus has been shown to increase the regeneration of liver cells, and protect them from inflammation. Many experiments with astragalus and liver disease consistently show that astragalus protects, repairs, and regenerates liver tissue damaged from a variety of toxic chemicals.[1-6]

One important area of concern with chronic liver disease is the development of scarring or cirrhotic tissue. When the liver is continually damaged, with chronic alcohol abuse for example, there begins a cascade of chemical responses to this damage. Liver cells that normally sleep (the quiescent state), called stellate cells, wake up. They wake up and immediately begin secreting scarring proteins. This creates very fibrous liver tissue. This fibrous tissue takes the place of previously normal cells and slowly begins to overwhelm the liver with massive scarring and loss of function. To help prevent this a medicine would have to interfere with this damaging process at the molecular level. Several research studies have found that astragalus does just that. It causes a shift in the chemistry of the liver. Large amounts of anti-inflammatory and antioxidant activity occurs, protecting against free radical damage. After administering astragalus, stellate cells go back to sleep and inflammation and liver destruction is significantly shut down.[7]

In a study of eighty-four people with advanced cirrhosis so serious that they began to develop moderate to severe hypertension, half the group received a placebo and half received astragalus combined with salvia, a type of sage. In the placebo group absolutely no improvement was seen. In the herbal combination group however, cirrhotic scarring slowed and hypertension reduced as well.[8] In study after study astragalus, by itself or combined with other herbs, was shown to prevent or significantly repair cirrhotic liver tissue.[9-16] This significant reduction of cirrhotic scarring is not achieved through synthetic medication. The standard medicine utilized for cirrhosis is actually synthetic bear bile, aka ursodiol. This synthetic medication is almost valueless in that it does not reduce mortality or liver transplantations. In fact, this medicine causes cancer in about one of every five people who have the liver disease called primary biliary cirrhosis. The not so funny joke I tell patients about this synthetic medicine is that it may not work well, but at least it is extremely expensive. Astragalus is much more effective, safer, and cheaper.

Endotoxins, as mentioned in the previous chapter, are chemicals secreted by certain bacteria, such as E. Coli. They are very damaging to our livers and can cause some of the most dangerous moments in infectious disease when a patient can be suddenly faced with life threatening liver organ failure. Studies with astragalus show that when mice are pretreated with astragalus polysaccharides they are protected from endotoxin induced liver damage via a strong antioxidant effect. Ultramicroscopic study showed that astragalus protects the very fragile liver mitochondria, the energy producing factories in our cells.[17] As wonderful as astragalus is in its ability to reduce endotoxin damage to our liver, it is best to not create this environment in the first place. Diets rich in whole grains, fruits, and vegetables create an environment that is not conducive to E. coli bacteria because they have less to eat, cannot tolerate an acid environment (although some pathogenic E. Coli species are developing an ability to exist in an acid pH environment), and are crowded out by fermentative bacteria such as Lactobacillus acidophilus. Probiotics such as Lactobacillus need much more attention from the medical community. They can potentially prevent and treat a variety of health problems.

Chronic Hepatitis B is a serious problem worldwide. Millions of people carry the virus chronically, and many more are infected temporarily. Several different drugs are utilized for chronic hepatitis B virus infection with minimal results. Physician researchers looking for an effective medicine to treat this difficult disease found that by adding astragalus to the drugs lamivudine and IFN alpha2b, a significant reduction of hepatitis virus could result.[18] Other studies on astragalus and hepatitis B have been very positive, with astragalus reducing Hepatitis B viral levels. Studies done at Shanghai Institute of Pharmaceutical Research showed that the saponin astragaloside IV may be the most potent anti-hepatitis compound found in astragalus.[19] In an experiment to see if astragalus could improve the effectiveness of hepatitis B vaccine, researchers found that the starches (polysaccharides) of astragalus significantly enhanced antibody formation, T cell proliferation, and increased dendritic cells to mature more rapidly.[20] This ability of astragalus to increase the effectiveness of several vaccines has been shown in multiple studies.[21,22]

Over the last twenty years I have received several phone calls from veterinarians asking for consultation regarding treating dogs that have ingested poisonous deathcap mushrooms (*Amanita phalloides*) while exploring the forest areas of California. This species of mushroom causes a significant destruction of both kidney and liver tissue. If not treated immediately, the outcome can be fatal. The most effective remedy combination for this life threatening event I have seen is astragalus combined with milk thistle (*Silymarin marianis*). Both of these herbs significantly protect and regenerate damaged liver and kidney tissue. I have never heard of any other health professional utilizing this life saving herbal combination. In this situation, these herbs are superheroes.

Chapter 9

LUPUS
SYSTEMIC LUPUS ERYTHEMATOSUS (SLE)

Lupus is an inflammatory disease where the body attacks itself. Being an autoimmune disease the present treatment for moderate to severe lupus is immune suppressive drugs. These drugs carry significant side effects often rivaling lupus in their damage. Different areas of the body are attacked in this disease, such as the heart, lungs, and kidneys. The kidneys often take the brunt of it. In severe lupus-caused infection and kidney damage, people often succumb to this overwhelming disease and die. Many articles, often written by people with little experience or knowledge of astragalus, warn against utilizing astragalus with lupus patients because they believe that astragalus will increase the autoimmune response and worsen lupus and its inflammation. All data to this date points to the opposite. Astragalus does not over amplify an immune system attack on tissues. It appears to enhance appropriate immune responses, reduces inflammation, and does not harm lupus sufferers.

Research on astragalus and lupus began in 1992 at the Chinese Air Force General Hospital. Twenty-eight patients with lupus were given astragalus to test their immune function. What was seen was that astragalus repaired a critical immune system defect common in people with lupus. Correcting this defect allowed for patients to normalize the production of natural killer cells. It did not overstimulate immune function.[1]

In an important study on lupus at the Shanghai University of Traditional Chinese Medicine, doctors studied 46 patients with lupus-caused kidney damage and infection. 23 patients received the immunosuppressive drug cyclophosphamide (Cytoxan) and 23 patients received cyclophosphamide plus astragalus. The results were startling. Simply adding astragalus to the common immunosuppressive therapy reduced the infection rate by 600%. The patients who received astragalus experienced increased kidney function and their red blood cell count increased as well. Immunosuppressive drugs lower white blood cell count significantly and in this study patients were protected from this drug side effect with astragalus. This simple addition of astragalus to their medication dramatically improved their kidney and blood cell health.[2]

In a study of eighty patients with lupus, researchers wanted to see if astragalus could keep lymphoctyes alive and functioning normally during immunosuppressive therapy. They were able to do both with astragalus.[3] One of the problems with lupus is that red blood cells become deformed and lose much of their oxygen carrying capacity. When scientists added astragalus to the blood of lupus patients they found that astragalus protected red blood cells, as well as white blood cells, from being damaged by the type of oxidation that occurs with lupus.[4] Other studies looking at lupus have found that astragalus helps normalize several immune system activities. These interesting studies lend credence to the idea that astragalus helps to normalize immune responses that include protecting tissue from the ravages of lupus. I could not characterize astragalus' effect on lupus better than the title of a 2008 research report, "Radix Astragali: a promising new treatment option for systemic lupus erythematosus".[5]

Chapter 10

AGING AND LIFE EXTENSION

In 20 years (or sooner) it is possible that the genetics and molecular mechanisms of human aging will be so well known and so well controlled that people will age at a much slower rate. It may become common to live well over 100 years. It is even possible that eventually human aging will slow down so much that death itself may be cheated. We are far from that in the second decade of the 21st century. But we are now beginning to understand many of the mechanisms that cause aging, as well as ways to slow down the clock. One aging mechanism that has received interest is in the area of oxidation. Antioxidants in foods have received much publicity in the last 20 years. Oxidation is merely the loss of an electron from atoms in our bodies tissues. Electrons are shaken lose or absorbed by other atoms that smash into them. As cells lose electrons they often die. Aging is merely cells dying faster than they can be replaced by healthy new cells. These lost electrons are picked up and used by other atoms. It is a normal part of metabolism, but a continual high oxidative state results in premature aging. Many environmental pollutants, cigarettes, and processed foods cause oxidation. Oxidation causes a loss of stem cells and progenitor cells that normally renew old or damaged tissue. Animals with fast metabolisms have increased rates of oxidation and that means their cells die faster and the animals die faster as well. Generally speaking, the smaller the animal and the faster its oxidation rate, the shorter its lifespan. There are some animals that live very long lives. The hard shell clam (*Artica*) for instance, lives more than 400 years in their very dark and cold water environment. In this environment, the clam's metabolic and oxidative rate is extremely slow. I still remember as a graduate student seeing pictures of chlorine factory workers from the early 20th century. Although the workers in the pictures were in their twenties and thirties, they looked 50 years older. Chlorine is an extremely potent oxidizer.

Astragalus has a reputation in Traditional Chinese Medicine for being an elixir for long life. It is only recently that research has showed how astragalus works as an anti-aging medicine. Firstly, astragalus as a potent antioxidant, extends the life and health of many cells.[1] The tissue that holds us together, called collagen, begins to age in our twenties and slowly loses its elasticity and begins to sag. Skin can age and sag due to oxidative stress primarily from ultraviolet rays from the sun. Ultraviolet A (UVA) is the worst of the energy frequencies that damage skin, resulting in what is called photoaging. Looking to see if astragalus could protect skin from UVA damage and aging, researchers at the Department of Dermatology at Jiangsu Hospital in China found that astragalus protects the skin by reducing chemicals that signal skin cells to die. Researchers working independently at Fudan University hospital came to the same conclusion and added that astragalus also inhibited the production of inflammatory NF kappaB.[2] Astragalus also reduces the production of MMP-1 and TIMP-1.[3] All three of these chemicals are not only associated with sunlight-induced skin damage and skin cell death, but are also responsible for the promotion of cancer. Studying the effects of ultraviolet B (UVB) sunlight, researchers found that astragalus also protects skin from damage and aging from UVB. Just like protection from UVA, astragalus reduces NF-kappaB and MMP-1 levels in skin cells (dermal fibroblasts) when they are stressed with UVB radiation. This significantly reduces the chances of developing sunburn induced skin cancer.[4]

Research done back in the early 1990's showed that when old rats were given astragalus their connective tissue not only stopped aging but in fact rejuvenated to an age comparable to young rats.[5] Astragalus could slow this aging mechanism in humans as well. In a series of studies at Peking University, scientists wanted to see if they could extend the life of human lung cells. In the experiment scientists, using an extract of astragalus called HDTIC, reported that they were able to significantly delay cell death, enhance cell growth, and increase antioxidant activity to levels seen only in young cells.[6-8] Astragalus was also tested to see if it could increase the amount of brain cells called M-cholinergic receptors. These receptors receive electrical stimulation and transmit it along brain pathways. As these receptors die of old age (oxidation), electricity cannot flow through brain tissue for clear thinking. This is the molecular version of the saying, "The lights are on, but nobody's home". Astragalus was able to increase the concentration of M-cholinergic receptors very significantly. This may translate to less brain senility.[9] Molecularly, the brain works much better and ages slower with the use of astragalus.

There has been much interest in the last twenty years over the energy factory of our cells, called the mitochondria. Mitochondria are responsible for manufacturing over 80% of our energy by making a chemical called ATP. ATP is often called the energy currency of our bodies. We spend a tremendous amount of this energy currency keeping cells alive and functioning efficiently. Many researchers theorize that if they could keep mitochondria alive and well, energy production would not fall off like it does now as we age. They believe that the mitochondria is a key to long and healthy life. While the mitochondria are manufacturing energy they also get bombarded by reactive oxygen species (ROS). These ROS chemicals are generated during energy creation and they leak in and around mitochondria, damaging and aging them with intense oxidation. Chinese researchers at the College of Life Sciences at Dalian National University looked to see if astragalus could slow down this mitochondria damage and aging. Utilizing a combination of the mineral iron and vitamin C they were able to cause huge damage to the mitochondrial membrane by what is called lipid peroxidation. Why does vitamin C, which is commonly known as an antioxidant, cause oxidation when mixed with iron? It is because vitamin C causes a change in iron's characteristics (called reduction) creating a powerful cell membrane oxidant. It does this efficiently in test tube experiments. In the human body iron-induced lipid peroxidation is not as significant. The main group to be concerned about with this are pregnant women who often take large doses of iron along with vitamin C to increase angiogenesis. The Dalian University researchers wanted to see if they could prevent and reverse this iron-caused oxidative damage to the mitochondrial membrane. What they found is that astragalus protects the mitochondria by sweeping up ROS, reducing the leakage of these toxic oxidant chemicals, and increasing production of several powerful antioxidants.[10]

To create new cells, our genetic code, called DNA, replicates itself over and over throughout our lifetime. Over time, it slowly loses some electrons and it begins to unravel its parts. Oxidation during DNA replication is highly responsible for our DNA being damaged and mutated. We have all seen what happens when you make a copy from a copy and continue with that exercise. The copies become poorer and poorer. Copying a paper may be relatively unimportant, but copying DNA is very important when perfectly intact DNA is needed to make healthy new cells.

Telomeres are protective caps on the ends of strands of DNA and they wear out and become shorter after many copies of cells are created over and over again. Right now there is a marketing frenzy going on over astragalus's purported ability to keep telomeres intact and thereby delivering perfect cell reproduction. One chemical isolated from astragalus and given the name TA65 (Telomerase Activation Sciences, Inc-65), is being studied as a silver bullet in aging. TA65 is derived from the astragaloside IV derivative cycloastragenol. Specifically targeting telomeres, the hope is that TA65 will keep the protective telomeres intact, thereby allowing for a perfect DNA copy from cell generation to generation. The theory being that if telomeres never fail in protecting and delivering undamaged DNA, we won't age as quickly (or at all) because every cell will be perfectly duplicated over and over. Research is limited and controversial.

A recent study at The National Cancer Center in Spain looked to see if telomeres could be protected with TA65. Success would be seen in a reduction of the shortening of telomeres. In fact in this study TA65 did increase average telomere length and decrease short telomeres. The mice used in the study had better glucose tolerance, reduced osteoporosis, and increased skin health. There was no cancer increase reported.[11] This is important because one of the mechanisms of cancer cell death is by shortening telomeres.[12,13] It has been a concern that generally increasing telomere length could keep cancer cells alive longer. For TA65 to work it must be proven not to enhance cancer cells survival. It's important to remember that this highly concentrated chemical TA65 does not contain the starches, astragalosides, isoflavonoids, or other chemicals found in astragalus that have been shown to prevent and slow cancer growth. At this point in time no one can be absolutely certain that TA65 will have this life extending effect without enhancing cancer cell lifespan. So far, astragalus derived TA65 has been shown to increase life span in laboratory mice without an increase in cancer.[14] It has also been shown to increase proliferation of human T cells, as well as enhance telomerase activity in those cells by up to 330%. Telomerase helps keep DNA intact by preventing telomeres from breaking down.[15] Aside from TA65, astragalus is effective in reducing random cellular aging and death through its antioxidant health promoting and tissue repairing effects.

Besides TA65, the astragalus chemical HDTIC mentioned previously has been shown to reduce the shortening of telomeres by one half as compared to controls. There was a large reduction in DNA damage, with improvement in DNA repair ability as well.[16] As interesting as these findings are, it is important to realize that telomeres are shortened by exposure to environmental pollutants such pesticides and other toxic chemicals throughout our lives.[17] We can reduce this shortening by limiting exposure to toxins, especially cigarettes and pesticides, and by having an antioxidant plant-based diet.

For those rare individuals interested in having their body frozen in liquid nitrogen after death with the hopes of being thawed out years later and cured of their life ending disease, astragalus may have something to offer this technology, called cryopreservation. Researchers at Southern Medical University in China harvested human fetal liver cells, added astragalus at various concentrations alone or combined with the antioxidant dimethylsulfoxide (DMSO) and froze them in liquid nitrogen for one month. The cells were thawed out in 30 days and checked for life and function. Results showed that Astragalus provided protection for these liver cells and was especially potent when combined with DMSO in this reanimation experiment.[18]

As much as we are interested in making life healthier and longer, it's just as important to know if Astragalus can help life begin. The problem of infertility is growing in the United States and around the world. In both men and women, fertility rates have dropped in the last twenty years and have only begun to slightly stabilize. Sperm is very fragile, and it's easily damaged and mutated by environmental toxins. There have been several studies looking at sperm health and astragalus's influence on sperm abnormalities. In a study at the Hainan Medical College in China, researchers wanted to see if astragalus could reduce the genetic damage to sperm from the toxic metal cadmium. Cadmium is a common environmental pollutant and can cause mutations, cancer, and cell death. In the study, astragalus increased sperm production and sperm count, and reduced cadmium-caused sperm mutations by 250%.[19]

In another study of infertile male volunteers, astragalus and five other herbs were tested to see if consuming them would increase the health and swimming ability (motility) of sperm. Of the six herbs tested, astragalus was the only one that increased sperm count and increased normal swimming of sperm. The infertile men were infertile no more.[20] In an experiment to see how astragalus protects sperm from the toxic chemotherapy chemical cyclophosphamide, researchers looked at several possible mechanisms. It was found that astragalus protected a critical chemical factor called CREM. CREM is a crucial gene regulator in the growing and maturing of sperm cells. In the experiment it was found that astragalus also increased sperm numbers and health.[21] Research with astragalus has shown that the herb dramatically increases sperm numbers and health, even in the face of environmental and drug toxins.

Chapter 11

HEALING INJURIES

After injury, our bodies have a remarkable ability to repair. We may not be able to regenerate large amounts of specialized tissue such as an opossum does when it regenerates a severed limb. But we do have a significant ability to heal. When an injury occurs, an inflammatory response begins which includes swelling, redness, heat, pain, and loss of function in the damaged area. Initially this response is helpful in protecting the damaged area from further injury. But if an injury is serious, and repair is slow and inefficient, the inflammatory response can continue for months or years. Damaged tissue does not repair efficiently during inflammation. The body will continually try to resolve the injury. If it can't efficiently heal the damage, the body's "plan B" is put into effect. Plan B is where the body fills in damaged tissue with loose connective tissue also known as scarring. This can result in a permanent injury. When this happens, the pain and loss of function continue and often become chronic for life. It is very important to heal injuries as swiftly and efficiently as possible so that this does not occur.

Astragalus can play an important role in healing damaged tissue. Firstly, astragalus increases the response to an injury. There is a significantly larger amount of healing activity that occurs at the damaged site when astragalus is utilized.[1] Astragalus increases growth factors at the site of injury, and these directly increase tissue repair.[2] Scientific studies consistently show that astragalus reduces the time in which injuries heal. Fractures, soft tissue injuries, and even nerve injuries have been studied. In each study very impressive results can be seen, with faster wound repair and reduced scarring.[3,4] Astragalus also enhances bone repair by speeding collagen growth to produce new bone tissue, as well as new blood vessels to the damaged bone.[5-7] This bone repairing effect can also be seen in the prevention and reversal of osteoporosis by astragalus and astragalus-based combinations.[8,9] The amount of new bone regeneration induced by astragalus was almost 400% more than controls in an experiment at the Central South University in China.[10] Possibly the most effective single component of astragalus for reversal of osteoporosis is astragaloside II. It has been shown to increase the proliferation and mineralization of osteoblasts, the cells that create bone tissue.[11]

Osteoporosis is a main concern for women after menopause or who have a total hysterectomy where the hormone producing ovaries are surgically removed along with the uterus. Astragalus may be of help in strengthening bone in these groups of women. In one study combining astragalus with dang gui (*Angelica sinensis*) and Epimedium herb, there was a significant increase in bone mineral density in lab animals.[12] In another study looking at combining astragalus with calcium, it was found that the combination of calcium supplementation and astragalus increased bone mineral density much better than using either one alone.[13] It appears that for anyone who takes calcium supplements for bone density it would be wise to take astragalus along with that calcium pill.

A formula mentioned previously in anemia chapter, dang gui bu xue tang, has also been traditionally used as a bone building formula. If it is to be utilized for bone repair and strength, it is vital that the dang gui in the formula is pre-cooked in wine before consumed. Many pills and powders of dang gui are prepared this way. There is a naturally occurring ingredient, ligustilide, that is found in raw dang gui. Ligustilide interferes with the availability and absorption of the astragalosides, polysaccharides, and isoflavonoids found in astragalus. If wine-cooked dang gui is added to astragalus, ligustilide is reduced, astragalus absorption is enhanced, and bone growth is increased.[14]

Noise-induced hearing loss is a problem for many Americans. Working or recreating in an environment that includes very loud noise can result in damage to the cochlea in the inner ear. Hearing loss and/or tinnitus (ringing) can begin immediately if the noise is loud enough or more commonly can occur gradually over months or years. If you have ever been to an event that is very loud and you leave with your ears ringing, you have experienced an acute and hopefully short term trauma to your inner ear. What's occurring in the inner ear during loud noise is that the tiny hair cells that line the inner ear become damaged by the generation of toxic chemicals that literally burnout this delicate tissue. Using electron microscopy to directly see the effects of loud noise on guinea pigs hearing, researchers found that significant free radical production was damaging the hair cells in the inner ear. They were interested to see if astragalus could prevent loud noise-induced hearing loss. Utilizing Astragaloside IV, one of the major constituents of astragalus root, they found that astragalus could stop the generation of free radicals and significantly reduce the damage to hair cells, thereby preventing hearing loss.[15] Seeing the biochemical mechanisms involved with lab animals, Dr. Xiong and his colleagues next tried to determine of astragalus could help in the recovery of acute loud noise trauma in humans. In their trial the average recovery of hearing and cessation of ear ringing (tinnitus) was significantly better after treatment with astragalus.[16] These preliminary studies could lead the way for more human trials that if duplicated could show that astragalus intake could reduce or even prevent and reverse loud noise induced hearing loss and tinnitus.

Even chemicals that slow down wound repair (called TIMP-1) are controlled and inhibited by astragalus, clearing the way for faster healing. In an experiment to see if astragalus could help heal serious nerve injuries, scientists at Chinese Changhua Christian Hospital used astragalus to see if large areas of nerve damage could be repaired. When a nerve is damaged and torn apart, very slow repair occurs, or the nerve scars and doesn't function at nearly the same capacity as an intact nerve does. Damaged nerves can generate serious pain. Working on sciatic nerve injuries of about one inch long, the researchers used silicone rubber chambers filled with astragalus and placed them in the one inch gap of damaged sciatic nerve tissue. It was hoped that astragalus could use this silicone frame and grow nerve tissue that would bridge this gap. At the end of the two month study, astragalus had increased the rate of healing significantly, with neurite growth, mylenation of axons, and total nerve area healing dramatically better than normally anticipated.[17]

Another interesting finding of astragalus is that it generally protects tissue from injury. Astragalus can make tissue stronger and less likely to be injured. If a person has astragalus in their bloodstream and is injured, that injury will have less chance of infection and greater chance for swift uncomplicated healing. This concept of strengthening tissue to reduce injury has been studied at length. For example, there is a procedure used to break down kidney stones called lithotripsy. Lithotripsy is a kind of high force ultrasound where very strong sound waves are used to break up kidney stones so that they can be eliminated though the urine. Originally marketed as a non-invasive safe therapy, it hasn't lived up to its hype. Unfortunately, lithotripsy can be very painful and the kidneys and other organs, such as the pancreas, are often damaged in this procedure. According to the National Institutes of Health, "Shock wave lithotripsy can cause vascular trauma to the kidneys and surrounding organs. This acute shock wave damage can be severe, can lead to scarring with a permanent loss of functional renal volume, and has been linked to potential serious long-term adverse effects. A recent retrospective study linking lithotripsy to the development of diabetes mellitus has further focused attention on the possibility that shock wave lithotripsy may lead to life-altering effects".[18]

In an experiment at the Chinese Institute of Urology, rabbits were given lithotripsy. One group served as normal controls and received no astragalus, and three groups each received either astragalus starches, or astragalus saponins, or astragalus flavonoids. Following the rabbits for two weeks, the scientists noted that the non-astragalus controls showed significant damage to kidney tissue caused by the lithotripsy. All three astragalus groups showed reduced levels of trauma-induced toxic chemical release. In the saponin and flavonoid groups, kidney damage was significantly milder than the untreated group, showing an important preventive effect with astragalus.[19] Eliminating kidney stones through lithotripsy is a procedure that causes acupuncturists like myself to both wince and feel somewhat self righteous. I have treated over 50 patients with kidney stones with acupuncture and herbs. All of them disintegrated and safely excreted disintegrated stones through the urine. Herbal formulas to deal with kidney stones have been developed by Chinese herb companies such as Mayway. Their herbal combination called Stone Formula works!

In a study to see if astragalus could reduce intestinal inflammation, astragalus was able to soothe inflamed intestinal tissue and create a normal gut environment. This could be seen at the genetic level. Astragalus inhibited the production of tumor necrosis factor-alpha and interleukin-8 through suppressing the p38 signaling pathway in gut tissue. These two compounds cause significant inflammatory responses. The importance cannot be overstated that astragalus affects disease at the most basic level of genetic expression.[20] Every known genetic and chemical mechanism that occurs in healing is positively influenced by astragalus. The bottom line is if an individual takes astragalus before or after an injury that person will enjoy more rapid healing.

Chapter 12

ASTRAGALUS AND INFLAMMATORY DISEASES

There are several other areas of astragalus research worth noting. Both osteoarthritis and rheumatoid arthritis have been studied. In a research project from Inha University in South Korea, researchers report that astragalus reversed inflammation and reduced joint damage in osteoarthritis.[1] In two animal studies of rheumatoid arthritis, astragalus reduced inflammation and synovial cell death.[2,3] More research needs to be done in the area of arthritis, but these preliminary studies are very encouraging. In my clinical practice, I have found that astragalus can allow a patient with advanced arthritis to significantly reduce intake of immune suppressive drugs. Astragalus reduces the toxicity and increases the efficacy of prednisone and other immune suppressive arthritis treatments.

In spite of our advances in medical technology, asthma is increasing around the world. Asthma deaths have never been higher than today. There are several synthetic medicine approaches to asthma. The first common strategy is to crush the immune system with immune lowering drugs such as prednisone, and second is to utilize the side effects of drugs that stimulates the fight or flight (sympathetic) response which includes dilation of the bronchial tubes. Neither one of these approaches is curative or healthy in the long run. Overuse of large amounts of prednisone-type medications opens up the patient to immune diseases such as cancer and multiple infections. Chronically revving up the nervous system with a sympathetic nervous system stimulant alters physiology dramatically. We are not designed to be in the fight or flight mode over a long period of time. This leads to reduced immune function, inflammation, altered sleep patterns, anxiety, and adrenal exhaustion.

What is needed is an approach that reduces the unhelpful immune response to pollens and other allergy promoting substances. Asthma is the body trying to shut off the inhalation of what it deems dangerous chemicals. Often they are not dangerous at all. What we need is the body to be reeducated. The goal is to utilize non-toxic medicines that gently alter the immune system to not just power down but to be more efficient at discerning between a real toxin and a harmless chemical such as pollen. Astragalus does just that. In two studies on asthma, researches wanted to see if astragalus could reduce the allergic asthma response to dust mites and other allergens. Astragalus reduced inflammation and allergy in both studies. In one of the studies astragalus was compared to an immune suppressive cortisone type drug. Both the astragalus and the immune suppressant drug worked well with the astragalus being just as effective with no side effects.[4,5] In laboratory mice with asthma, astragalus was able to reduce overproduction of eosinophils, an immune cell created during allergy response. It was also shown to normalize other inflammatory chemicals as well, including certain interleukins.[6] In another laboratory study, astragalus significantly reduced asthma signs and symptoms. The researchers in this study concluded, "Our results indicated that it (astragalus) should be used as a supplementary therapy on preventing asthma attacks in chronic asthma patients".[7] The latest studies show that astragalus reduces asthma at the genetic level and that measurements of this inflammatory gene reduction are quite significant.[8]

Aside from allergic asthma, allergic rhinitis or "hay fever" affects millions of Americans each year. In a 6 week, double-blind placebo-controlled study of 48 adult patients with moderate to severe allergies, an astragalus-based food supplement popular in eastern Europe called HMC (herb and mineral complex) was tested to see if it would reduce symptoms such as rhinitis (runny nose) and increase quality of life. Patients reported significant improvement in general health, quality of health, and significant reduction of all symptoms of hay fever.[9]

Astragalus may assist in reducing skin inflammatory diseases. In an early trial with astragalus versus allergic dermatitis, astragalus was able to reverse the inflammatory response and significantly decrease skin inflammation.[10] Researchers at the University of

Valencia in Spain found that astragalus reduces the inflammatory chemical 5-lipoxygenase, which is involved in promoting psoriasis and eczema.[11] Skin diseases were one of the main focuses of the first book written 1,000 years ago that describes astragalus and its medicinal value.

Astragalus and Optimal Health

As we can see astragalus is extremely helpful in preventing and successfully treating a wide variety of serious injuries and diseases. Astragalus could be called the "great augmenter" in that it increases the efficiency of many medications, while often reducing their side effects. Astragalus also increases the health of many important organ systems. As such, the opportunity to increase general health is available to almost everyone who takes Astragalus as part of a health building lifestyle. Astragalus will not save a person from themselves if poor lifestyle choices are a constant. If a person is interested in doing the work necessary for optimal health, astragalus can make a positive difference. Increased energy, improved immune function, enhanced physiological efficiency, swifter healing, and a general feeling of well being can be achieved by taking Astragalus.

USING ASTRAGALUS

Astragalus is generally needed in moderate to large amounts to be optimally effective. In the very few studies that have not shown astragalus to be helpful there is a pattern of the researchers using very low doses. An example is a Japanese study on childhood asthma. In that study researchers gave children an herbal combination that only included about 125 milligrams of astragalus per dose. This is 10 to 30 times less than is utilized for children in clinical settings. The researchers were very critical of astragalus, stating that parents should look elsewhere for an effective medicine. But as you can see they were naïve when it comes to understanding astragalus and its dosage requirements. To get the most from astragalus it would be best to find an herbalist, acupuncturist, doctor of oriental medicine, naturopath (only graduates from an accredited naturopathic college), or the rare medical doctor who is competent in the area of herbal therapy. That way you can be guided to using astragalus by itself or combined with other herbs and natural treatments that will enhance your chances for success.

Astragalus is available to consumers in many forms. The most basic is as a cut whole root. The roots are usually cut length wise, and resemble a wooden tongue depressor. You may also see them as short slices.

-Root pieces are simmered in water for 20 to 40 minutes to extract the ingredients within the woody roots. Since roots vary in size, it is difficult to recommend an exact amount. In general, three to six root slices simmered in 12-16 ounces of water constitute a single dose. These slices make wonderful additions to soups and teas.

-Crude crushed astragalus powder: 1000-5000 mg. per dose. One to three doses per day.

-Concentrated powder/capsule: 1000-3000 mg. One to three times per day. There are significant differences in concentrations of astragalus. Some companies offer 5:1 or even 15:1 concentrations. Other companies offer astragalus in its standardized form. This should be listed on the label as, "contains 0.5% of hydroxy-3-methoxy-isoflavone-7".

Astragalus polysaccharides, saponins, and isoflavonoids are also commercially available individually. These extracts often reflect concentrated astragalus utilized in research. They are many times stronger than astragalus root themselves and are only advised to be taken under supervision of a knowledgeable herbal expert.

Astragalus-based combinations have been a hallmark of traditional herbal medicine for hundreds of years. As good as Astragalus is by itself, its ability to help other herbs, as well as many synthetic medications work more effectively, makes it a wonderful candidate for combination therapy. Board certified acupuncturists and experienced herbalists can combine astragalus with other herbs to create customized formulas to fit individual patients needs. Here are a few classic traditional Chinese medicine formulas. Formulas are very specific in terms of who and what they treat.

Bu Zhong Yi Qi Wan
Astragalus, Codonopsis, Atractylodes, Glycyrrhiza, Angelica sinensis, Cimicifuga, Bupleurum, Citrus reticulata, Zingiber officinale

This classic formula is one of the more popular combinations in traditional Chinese medicine. It is designed to tonify the vital energy in the body called Qi (pronounced:chee). It increases resistance to disease, strengthens the connective tissues, and improves digestion. Often used when one is recovering from long illness, this formula is very rejuvenating.

Dang Gui Bu Xue Tang
Mentioned in the text for anemia, leukopenia, bone repair, and brain health, this is a classic simple formula of astragalus and dang gui. The ratio of the herbs has been studied extensively. Doctors of Oriental medicine often utilize four to one or five to one ratios of astragalus to dang gui. As mentioned in the anemia chapter, several studies have shown that the 5:1 ratio is the most effective for building both red and white blood cells.

Shen Qi Da Bu Wan
Astragalus and Codonopsis root

This simple combination of these two health building herbs is often used for general health, to recover from long illness including cancer therapy, and chronic fatigue syndrome. Codonopsis is sometimes called the poor persons ginseng because it has some of the health building qualities of ginseng without the high price tag.

Shen Qi Wu Wei Zi Wan
Astragalus, Schizandra, Codonopsis, and Wild Jujube seed

This formula is the previous combination with the addition of two herbs, schizandra and wild jujube seeds. Schizandra (pronounced *skiz AND drah*) is becoming more popular in the west. It has impressive health building qualities. It is astringent and stops spontaneous sweating from fatigue. A large amount of studies have shown that this herb heals liver tissue. The wild jujube seeds are relaxing and stress reducing, and several studies have shown health building effects, especially for the liver. By adding these two herbs this formula becomes both an anti-stress and health rejuvenating combination.

Huang Qi He Shou Wu Wan
Astragalus, He Shou Wu (*Polygonum multiflorum/Reynoutria multiflora*), Jujube dates, and Codonopsis

This health promoting formula was prescribed to me by Michael Broffman, the well respected traditional Chinese medicine practitioner, in 1979 when I was a naturopathic medical student recovering from chronic fatigue. It is a very valuable illness recovery and health building formula that includes He shou wu, a legendary and powerful herb that deserves a book written about it.

Bu Fei Wan
Astragalus, Rehmannia, Morus alba, Aster tataricus, Changium mymoiodes root, Schisandra, and Panax ginseng

This formula is specifically utilized for astragalus's lung tonic purposes. It is very helpful for people with weak lung function including asthma, chronic obstructive pulmonary disease (COPD), and persistent or recurring bronchitis.

Yu Ping Feng Wan
Astragalus, Atractylodes, and Saposhnikovia

Known commonly as Jade Screen Teapills, this formula has one of the largest concentrations (often over 60%) of astragalus. It is well known for its adaptogenic and immune system building abilities. The most common usage is to prevent infections such as influenza and common colds. It is mentioned in the text as a preventive against toxin-induced liver inflammation and scarring.

Recommended Herb Companies
Mayway Corporation

I have a long history with Mayway. When they were just a single store in San Francisco in the 1980's, I would buy herbs from May Lau who owned this wonderful Chinese herb shop. May's children, would assist her with orders at the store. I still think of them, smiling, helpful, humble kids, always ready to help their mom. These children are now adults and have succeeded in creating the largest American-based Chinese herbal medicine company in the world. They have excellent customer service and are environmentally and socially caring people. Their herbs are of very high quality. Mayway is unique in that they oversee herb sourcing, extraction, processing, bottling, and distribution of their herbs. No other Chinese herb company I have seen can compete with Mayway quality. They deserve the success they have nurtured.

Mayway Corp.
1338 Mandela Parkway
Oakland, Ca. 94607
www.mayway.com
1-800-MAYWAY(262-9929)

Herb Pharm

Herb Pharm is another company I have utilized for a very long time. I still remember Ed Smith, co-founder of Herb Pharm, pulling up to my naturopathic college with his jeep in the late 1970's. Appearing like a patent medicine salesman of the 19th century, Ed would open up the back and proudly display his outstanding herbal wares. Herb Pharm has come a long way since then. They are a much larger company now. They still create very high standard herbal products, including a wonderful astragalus tincture.

Herb Pharm
P.O. Box 116
Williams, Or. 97544
www.herb-pharm.com
800-328-4372

Horizon Herb Seed Company

This is the best herb seed company I have seen. They carry a very large variety of both western and eastern herbs. The owners, Richo and Sena Cech, have continually expanded their interesting catalog. Great people, great products.

Horizon Herbs
PO Box 69
Williams, Or. 97544
www.horizonherbs.com
541-846-6704

There are several other herb companies offering good to excellent quality astragalus. They include Crain Herbs, Gaia Herbs, Sun Ten, Frontier Natural Products Coop, and Oregon Wild Harvest.

REFERENCES

Chapter 1 - What is Astragalus?

1. Qian D, Chen M, et al. A taxonomic study on the original plant of radix astragali. *Yao Xue Xue Bao (Acta Pharmaceatica Sinica)*. 2009 Dec;44(12):1429-33.

2. Sun H, Guan S, Huang M. Study on new extraction technology of astragaloside IV. *Zhong Yao Ca (Journal of Chinese Medicinal Materials)*. 2005;28(8):705-8.

3. Wang DQ, Shen WM, et al. The effect of honey-frying on anti-oxidation activity of Astragalus mongholicus. *Zhongguo Zhong Yao Za Zhi (China Journal of Chinese Materia Medica)*. 1994;Mar,19(3);150-2,190.

4. Tian YH, Jin FY, Lei H. Effects of processing on contents of saccharides in huangqi (Astragalus). *Zhongguo Zhong Yao Za Zhi (China Journal of Chinese Materia Medica)*. 2003 Feb;28(2):128-9, 173.

5. Hao GJ, Zhang K, et al. RT-qPCR analysis of dexB and galE gene expression of Streptococcus alactolyticus in Astragalus membranaceus fermentaion. *Applied Microbiology and Biotechnology.* 2013 Apr. 9 e-pub.

6. Rosenbleuth M, Martinez-Romero E. Bacterial endophytes and their interactions with hosts. *Molecular Plant-Microbe Interactions*. 2006;19:827-837.

7. Ryan RP, Germaine K, et al. Bacterial endophytes: recent developments and applications. *FEMS Microbiology Letters* 2008;278:1-9.

8. Sun H, Guan S, Huang M. Study on new technology of astragaloside IV. *Zhong Yao Cao (Journal of Chinese Medicinal Materials).* 2005 Aug;28(8):705-8.

9. Han QB, Song JZ, et al. Preparative isolation of cyclolanostane-type saponins from Astragalus membranaceus (Bge.) Var. mongholicus (Bge.) Hsiao by TLC-MS/MS guided high-speed counter-current chromatography. *Journal of Separation Science.* 2007 Jan;30(1):135-40.

10. Yu QT, Qi LW, et al. Determinaton of seventeen main flavonoids and saponins in the medicinal plant Huang qi (Radix astragali) by HPLC-DAD-ELSD. *Journal of Separation Science*. 2007 June;30(9): 12920-9.

11. Wang D, Song Y, et al. Simultaneous analysis of seven astragalosides in Radix Astragali and related preparations by liquid chromatography coupled with electrospray ionization time-of-flight mass spectrometry. *Journal of Separation Science*. 2006 Aug;29(13):2012-22.

12. Kim JS, Yean MH, et al. Two new cycloartane saponins from the roots of Astragalus membranaceus. *Chemical and Pharmaceutical Bulletin (Tokyo)*. 2008 Jan;56(1):105-8.

13. Yan MM, Chen CY. Enhanced extraction of astragalosides from Radix Astragali by negative pressure cavitation-accelerated enzyme pretreatment. *Bioresource Technology.* 2010 Oct;101(19):7462-71

14. Xia GP, Liu P, Han YM. Determination of the total astragaloside IV in Radix Astragali. *Zhong Yao Cai (Journal of Chinese Medicinal Materials).* 2008 Mar;31(3):385-7.

15. Liu M, Zhou J, et al. Amic solution hydrolysis for improving content of astragaloside IV in extract of Radix Astragali. *Zhongguo Zhong Yao Za Zhi (China Journal of Chinese Materia Medica).* 2008 Mar;33(6):635-8.

16. Wang ZP, Gao Y, et al. Study on purification of total flavonoids and saponins of Astragalus with macroporous resin. *Zhong Yao Cai (Journal of Chinese Materia Medica).* 2010 Jul;33(7):1163-6.

17. Liu J, Yang H, et al. Comparative study of wild and cultivated astragali radix in Daqingshen district of Wuchuan of Neimenggu. *Zhongguo Yao Za Zhi (China Journal of Chinese Materia Medica).* 2011 June;36(12):1577-81.

18. Song JZ, Yiu HH, et al. Chemical comparison and classification of Radix Astragali by determination of isoflavonoids and astragalosides. *Journal of Pharmaceutical and Biomedical Analysis.* 2008 June 9;47(2):399-406.

19. Xu RY, Nan P, et al. Ultraviolet irradiation induces accumulation of isoflavonoids and transcription of genes of enzymes involved in the calycosis-7-0-beta-d-glucoside pathway in Astragalus membranaceus Bge. Var mongholicus (Bge.) Hsiao. *Physiologia Plantarum.* 2011 July;142(3):265-73.

20. Song Y, Lip, et al. Micellar electrokinetic chromatography for the quantitative analysis of flavonoids in the radix of Astragalus membranaceus var. mongholicus. *Planta Medica.* 2008 Jan;74(1):84-9.

21. Xiao HB, Krucker M, et al. Determination and identification of isoflavonoids in Radix astragali by matrix solid-phase dispersion extraction and high-performance liquid chromatography with photodiode array and mass spectrometric detection. *Chromatography.* 2004 Apr 2;1032(1-2)117-24.

22. Lu YW, et al. Identification and determination of flavonoids in astragali radix by high performance liquid chromatography coupled with DAD and ESI-MS detection. *Molecules.* 2011 March 9;16(3) 2293-2303.

23. Yu DH, Bao Ym, et al. Studies of chemical constituents and their antioxidant activities from Astragalus mongholicus Bunge. *Biomedical and Environonmental Sciences.* 2005 Oct;18(5):297-301.

24. Li SL, Gu X, et al. Correlation studies of contents of copper and organic components in astragalus roots. *Zhongguo Zhong Yao Za Zhi (China Journal of Chinese Materia Medica).* 2006 Aug:Aug;31(15):1249-53.

25. Wang WL, Liang ZS, et al. . Determination of mineral elements in different parts of Astragalus membranaceus (Fisch.) by FAAS. *Guang Pu Xue Yu Guang Pu Fen Xi.* 2008 May;28(5):1168-71.

26. Lei LD, Ouyang L, et al. Character study of content and correlativity of elements in Radix Astragali obtained from different regions. *Zhongguo Zhong Yao Za Zhi (China Journal of Chinese Materia Medica).* 2008 Feb;33(3):255-8.

27. Jin S, Li P, et al. Determination of active components in Radix astragali and its medicinal preparations by capillary electrophoresis with electrochemical detection. *Se Pu (Chinese Journal of Chromatography).* 2009 Mar;27(2):229-32.

28. Sun H, Xie D, et al. Study on the relevance between beany flavor and main bioactive components in Radix Astragali. *Journal of Agricultural and Food Chemistry.* 2010 May 12;58(9):4458-73.

29. Wang WL, Wang Z, Xu FL. Effects of nitrogen, phosphorus and potassium application on growth and active ingredients of Astragalus membranaceus. *Zhonguo Zhong Yao Za Zhi (China Journal of Chinese Materia Medica).* 2008 Aug;33(15):1802-1806.

30. Zhang WJ, Wojta J, Binder BR. Regulation of the fibrolynic potential of cultured human umbilical vein endothelial cells: astragaloside IV downregulates plasminogen activator inhibitor-1 and upregulates tissue-type plaminogen activator expression. *Journal of Vascular Research.* 1997;34:273-280.

31. Yin XJ, Liu DX, et al. A study on the mutagenicity of 102 raw pharmaceuticals used in Chinese traditional medicine. *Mutation Research.* 1991 May;260(1):73-82.

32. Wang DQ, Tian YP, et al. Anti-mutagenesis effects of total flavonoids of Astragalus. *Zhongguo Zhong Yao Za Zhi (China Journal of Chinese Materia Medica).* 2003 Dec:28(12):1164-7.

33. Braun K, Romero J, et al. Production of swainsonine by fungal endophytes of locoweed. *Mycological Research.* 2003 Aug;107(Pt8):980-8.

34. Ralphs MH, Creamer R, et al. Relationship between the endophyte Embellisia spp. and the toxic alkaloid swainsonine in major locoweed species (Astragalus and Oxytropis). *Journal of Chemical Ecology.* 2008 Jan:34(1):32-8.

35. Ralphs MH, James LF. Locoweed grazing. *Journal of Natural Toxins.* 1999 Feb;(1):47-51.

36. Galeas ML, Zhang LH, et al. Seasonal fluctuations of selenium and sulfur accumulation in selenium hyperaccumulators and relate nonaccumulators. *New Phytology*. 2007;173(3):517-25.

37. El Mehdawi AF, Cappa JJ, et al. Interactions of selenium hyperaccumulators and nonaccumulators during cocultivation on seleniferous or nonseleniferous soil-the importance of good neighbors. *New Phytology*. 2012, Jan 23.

38. Pao LH, Hu OY, et al. Herb-drug interaction of 50 Chinese herbal medicines on CYP3A4 activity in vitro and vivo. *American Journal of Chinese Medicine*. 2012;40(1):57-73.

39. Zhang YD, Shen JP, et al. Effects of astragalus (ASI, SK) on experimental liver injury. *Yao Xue Xue Bao (Acta Pharmaceutica Sinica)*.1992;27(6):401-6.

Chapter 2 - Diabetes

1. Cavallo MG, Fava D, et al. Increased frequency of IgM antibodies to cow's milk proteins in Hungarian children with newly diagnosed insulin-dependent diabetes: implications for disease pathogenesis. *Lancet*. 1996;348:926-928.

2. Karjalainen J, Martin J, et al. A bovine albumin peptide as a possible trigger of insulin-dependent diabetes. *New England Journal of Medicine*. 1992;327:302-307.

3. Saukkonen T, Savilahti E, et al. Increased frequency of IgM antibodies to cow's milk proteins in Hungarian children with newly diagnoses insulin-dependent diabetes mellitus. *European Journal of Pediatrics*. 1996;155:885-889.

4. Campbell TC, Campbell TM. Autoimmune Diseases, Type 1 Diabetes. *The China Study*. 187-192. Benbella Books. 2006.

5. Mijac V, Arrieta J, et al. Role of environmental factors in the development of insulin-dependent diabetes mellitus (IDDM) in insulin-dependent Venezuelan children. *Investigacion Clinica*. 1995;36:73-82.

6. Head K. Type 1 diabetes: Prevention of the disease and its complications. *Alternative Medicine Reviews*. 1997;2(4):256-281.

7. United States Department of Agriculture. Economic Research Service. *Agriculture Fact Book*. 2001.Chapter 2, Pg. 20.

8. Crawford MA, Marsh D. *Nutrition and Evolution*. New Caanan, Ct:Keats Publishing;1995.

9. Gilbert RL, Mielke JH, eds. *The Analysis of Prehistoric Diets*. Orlando, Fl: Academic Press: 1985.

10. Eaton SB, Eaton SB III, et al. An evolutionary perspective enhances understanding of human nutritional requirements. *Journal of Nutrition.* 1996:126:1732-1740.

11. Eaton SB, Eaton SB III, Konner MJ. Paleolithic nutrition revisited: a twelve year retrospective on its nature and implications. *European Journal of Clinical Nutrition.* 1997;51:207-216.

12. www.cdc.gov/NCCDPHP/dch/multimedia/infographics.htm

13. Rich, SS. Genetics of diabetes and its complications. *Jamaican Society of Nephrology.* 17:353-360, 2006.

14. Navarro-Gonzales JF, Mora-Fernandez C. The role of inflammatory cytokines in diabetic nephropathy. *Journal of the American Society of Nephrology.* 2008 Mar 1.Vol. 19:3 433-442.

15. Tesch GH. MCP-1/CCL2: A new diagnostic marker and therapeutic target for progressive renal injury in diabetic nephropathy. *American Journal of Physiology-Renal Physiology.* 2008 April;294(4):697-701.

16. Li M, Wang W, et al. Meta-analysis of the clinical value of Astragalus membranaceus in diabetic nephropathy. *Journal of Ethnopharmacology.* 2011 Jan 27;133(2):412-9.

17. Zhang J, Xie X, et al. Systemic review of the renal protective effect of Astragalus membranaceus root on diabetic nephropathy in animal models. *Journal of Ethnopharmacology.* 2009 Nov 12;126(2):189-96.

18. Hong XP, Zhang XZ, et al. Effect of Astragalus mongholicus on renal gene expression in mice with diabetic nephropathy. *Zhongguo Zhong Yao Za Zhi (China Journal of Chinese Materia Medica).* 2008 Mar;33(6):675-80.

19. Zhang YW, Wu CY, et al. Merit of Astragalus polysaccharides in the improvement of early diabetic nephropathy with an effect on mRNA expressions of NF-kappaB and I-kappaB in renal cortex of streptozotoxin-induced diabetes. *Journal of Ethnopharmacology.* 2007 Dec 3;114(3):387-92.

20. Chen W, Li YM, Yu MH. Astragalus polysacchrides inhibited diabetic cardiomyopathy in hamsters depending on suppression of heart chymase activation. *Journal of Diabetes Complications.* 2010 May-June;24(3):199-208.

21. Chen W, Yu MH, et al. Beneficial effects of astragalus polysaccharide treatment of heart chymase activities and cardiomyopathy in diabetic hamsters. *Acta Diabetologica.* 2010 Dec;47(suppl 1):35-46.

22. Liu KZ, Li JB, et al. Effects of astragalus and saponins of Panax notoginseng on MMP-9 in patients with type two diabetic microangiopathy. *Zhongguo Zhong Yao Za Zhi (China Journal of Chinese Materia Medica)*. 2004 Mar;29(3):264-6.

23. Chen W, Li YM, Yu MH. Effects of Astragalus polysaccharides on chymase, angiotensin-converting enzyme, and angiotensis II in diabetic cardiomyopathy in hamsters. *Journal of Internal Medicine Research*. 2007 Nov-Dec;35(6):873-7.

24. Li C, Cao L, Zeng Q. Astragalus prevents diabetic rats from developing cardiomyopathy by downregulating angiotensin II type 2 receptors expression. *Journal of Huazhong University, Science and Technological Medical Science*. 2004;24(4):379-84.

25. Sanchez A, Reeser JL, et al. Sugars in human neutrophilic phagocytosis. *American Jounal of Clinical Nutrition*. 1973. Nov;26(11):1180-4.

26. Zhou X, Xu Y, et al. Increased galectin-1 expression in muscle of astragalus polysaccharide-treated Type 1 diabetic mice. *Journal of Natural Medicine*. 2011 Jul;65(3-4):500-507.

27. Li RJ, Qiu SD, et al. The immunotherapeutic effects of Astragalus polysaccharide in type 1 diabetic mice. *Biological and Pharmaceutical Bulletin*. 2007 Mar;30(3):470-6.

28. Li RJ, Qiu SD. Immunomodulatory effects of Astraglus polysaccharide in diabetic mice. *Journal of Chinese Integrative Medicine*. 2008 Feb;6(2), 166-170.

29. Li CD, Li JJ, et al. Inhibitory effect of Astragalus polysaccharides on apoptosis of pancreatic beta-cells mediated by Fas in diabetes mellitus rats. *Zhong Yao Cai (Journal of Chinese Medicinal Materials)*. 2011 Oct;34(10):1579-82.

30. Tang D, He B, et al. Inhibitory effects of two major isoflavonoids in Radix Astragali on high glucose-induced mesangial cells proliferation and AGEs-induced endothelial cells apoptosis. *Planta Medica*. 2011 May;77(7):729-32.

31. Xu Y, Feng L, et al. Calycosin protects HUVECs from advanced glycation end products-induced macrophage infiltration. *Journal of Ethnopharmacology*. 2011 Sep1;137(1);359-70.

32. Qin Q, Niu J, et al. Astragalus membranaceus inhibits inflammation via phospho-p38 mitogen activated protein kinase(MAPK) and nuclear factor(NF)-kB pathways in advanced glycation end product-stimulated macrophages. *International Journal of Molecular Science*. 2012;13(7):8379-87.

33. Motomura K, Fujiwara Y, et al. Astragalosides isolated from the root of astragalus radix inhibit the formation of advanced glycation end products.

Journal of Agriculture Food Chemistry. 2009. Sep 9:57(17);7666-72.

34. Lau TW, Sahota DS, et al. An in vivo investigation on the wound-healing effect of two medicinal herbs using an animal model with foot ulcer. *European Surgery Research.*2008;41(1):15-23.

35. Lau TW, Chan YW, et al. Radix astragli and radix rehmanniae, the principal components of two antidiabetic foot ulcer formulae, elicit viability-promoting effects on primary fibroblasts cultured from diabetic foot ulcer tissue. *Phytotherapy Research.* 2009 June;23(6):809-15.

36. Tam JC, Lau KM, et al. The in vivo and in vitro diabetic wound healing effects of a 2-herb formula and its mechanisms of action. *Journal of Ethnopharmacology.* 2011 Apr 12;134(3):831-8.

37. Lai PK, Chan JY, et al. Isolation of anti-inflammatory fractions and compounds from the root of Astragalus membranaceus. *Phytotherapy Research.* 2012 June 13. Doi: 10. 1002/ptr.4759 Epub.

38. Wang Y, Zhu Y, et al. Formononetin attenuates IL-1beta-induced apoptosis and NF-kB activation in INS-1 cells. *Molecules.* 2012 Aug 24;17(9):10052-64.

39. Li FL, Li X, et al. Astragaloside IV downregulates beta-catenin in rat keratinocytes to counter LiCl-induced inhibition of proliferation and migration. *Evidence Based Complementary and Alternative Medicine.* 2012;2012:956107. Epub 2012 May 28.

40. Zhang Q, Wei F, et al. Transcriptional profiling of human fibroblast cell line Hs induced by herbal formula Astragali Radix and Rehmanniae Radix. *Journal of Ethnopharmacology.* 2011 Dec 8;138(3):668-75.

41. Xu A, Wang H, et al. Selective elevation of adipinectin production by the natural compounds derived from a medicinal herb alleviates insulin resisitance and glucose intolerance in obese mice. *Endocrinology.* 2009 Feb;150(2):625-33.

42.Zou F, Mao XQ, et al. Astragalus polysaccharides alleviate glucose toxicity and restores glucose homeostasis in diabetic states via activation of AMPK. *Acta Pharmacologica Sinica.* Dec;30(12):1607-15.

43. Lui M, Wu K, et al. Astragalus polysaccharide improves insulin sensitivity in KKAy mice: regulation of PKB/GLUT4 signaling in skeletal muscle. *Journal of Ethnopharmacology.* 2010 Jan 8;127(1):32-7.

44. Jiang B, Yang Y, et al. Astragaloside IV attenuates lipolysis and improves insulin resistance induced by TNF-alpha in 3T3-L1 adipocytes. *Phytotherapy Research.* 2008 Nov;22(11):1434-9.

45. Zhang DM, Lou LX, et al. Effects of astragalus membranaceus and potentilla discolor mixture on insulin resistance and its related mRNA expressions in KKAy mice with type 2 diabetes. *Zhong Xi Yi Jie He Xue Bao (Journal of Chinese Integrative Medicine)*.2012. July;10(7):821-6.

46. Yu J, Zhang Y, et al. Inhibitory effects of astragaloside IV on diabetic peripheral neuropathy in rats. *Canadian Journal of Physiology and Pharmacology.* 2006 June;84(6):579-87.

47. Hammes HP, Lin J, et al. Pericytes and the pathogenesis of diabetic retinopathy. *Diabetes.* 2002 51 (10): 3107-12.

48. Cheng L, Zhang G, et al. Systemic review and meta-analysus of 16 randomized clinical trials of radix astragali and its prescriptions for diabetic retinopathy. *Evidence Based Complementary and Alternative Medicine.* 2013;2013:762783. Mar 21.

49. Gao D, Guo Y, et al. An aqueous extract of Radix astragali, Angelica sinensis, and Panax notoginseng is effective in preventing diabetic retinopathy. *Evidence-Based Complementary and Alternative Medicine.* 2013;2013:578165. Epub.

Chapter 4 - Immunity

1. Wang RT, Shan BE, Li QX. Extracorpeal experimental study on immunomodulatory activity of Astragalus membranaceus extract. *Zhongguo Zhong Xi Yi Jei He Za Zhi (Chinese Journal of Integrated Traditional and Western Medicine).* 2002 June;22(6):453-6.

2. Gao QT, Cheung JK, et al. A Chinese herbal decoction, Dangui Buxue Tang, prepared from Radix Astragali and Radix Angelica Sinensis, stimulates the immune responces. *Planta Medica.* 2006 Oct;72(13):1227-31.

3. Zhuge ZY, Zhu YH, et al. Effects of astragalus polysaccharide on immune response of porcine PBMC stimulated with PRRSV or CSFV. *PLoS One (Public Library of Science One).* 2012;7(1):e29320 Epub 2012 Jan 9.

4. Zhao LH, Ma ZX, et al. Characteristics of polysaccharides from Astragalus radix as the macrophage stimulator. *Cellular Immunology.* 2011 Aug 25;271(2):329-34.

5. Ning KJ, Ruan XC, et al. Effects of Huangqi on phagocytic activity of peritoneal macrophage of mice. *Zhongguo Zhong Yao Za Zhi (China Journal of Chinese Materia Medica).* 2005 Nov;30(21):1670-2.

6. Zhao S, Zhang WH, et al. Effects of Astragalus polysaccharides and Cordyceps sinensis mycelium mixture on the transforming growth factor-beta 1 expression

in chronic rejection of artery transplantation: experiment with rats. *Zhonghua Yi Xue Za Zhi*. 2007 Mar 27;87(12):851-4.

7. Qu LL, Su YL, et al. Astragalus membranaceus injection delayed allograph survival related with CD4 CD25 regulatory T cells. *Transplantation Proceedings.* 2010 Nov. 3793-97

8. Clement-Kruzel S, Hwang SA, et al. Immune modulation of macrophage pro-inflammatory response by goldenseal and Astragalus extracts. *Journal of Medical Foods.* 2008 Sep;11(3)493-8.

9. Wang Z, Cheng Z, Fang X. Antiviral action of combined use of rhizoma Polygoni cuspidate and radix Astragali on HSV-1 strain. *Zhongguo Zhong Yao Za Zhi (China Journal of Chinese Materia Medica).* 1999 Mar;24(3):176-80, 192.

10. Yang X, Huang S, et al. Evaluation of the adjuvant properties of Astragalus membranaceus and Scutellaria baicalensis in the immune protection induced by UV-attenuated Toxoplasma gondii in mouse models. *Vaccine.* 2010 Jan 8;28(3):737-43.

11. Liu WJ, Liu B, et al. Influence of ganciclovir and astragalus membranaceus on proliferation of hematopoietic progenitor cells of cord blood after cytomegalovirus infection in vitro. *Zhonghua Er Ke Za Zhi (Chinese Journal of Pediatrics).* 2004 July;42(7):490-4.

12. Lee JH, Lee JY, et al. Immunoregulatory activity by daucosterol, a beta-sisterol glycoside, induces protective Th1 immune response against disseminated Candidiasis in mice. *Vaccine.* 2007 May 10;25(19):3834-40.

13. Zhang XL, YU XH, et al. Prophylactic immunization of dangguibuxue decoction against Cryptosporidium infection in immune suppressed mice. *Zhongguo Ji Sheng Chong Xue Yu Ji Sheng Chong Bing Za Zhi (Chinese Journal of Parasitology and Parasite Diseases).* 2008 June30;26(3):179-82.

14. Niu GH, Sun X, Zhang CM. Effect of compound astragalus recipe on lymphocyte subset, immunoglobulin and complements in patients with myasthenia gravis. *Zhongguo Zhong Xi Yi Jie He Za Zhi (Chinese Journal of Integrated Traditional and Western Medicine).* 2009 Apr;29(4):305-8.

15. Xu HD, You CG, et al. Effects of Astragalus polysaccharides and astragalosides on the phagocytosis of Mycobacterium tuberculosis by macrophages. *Journal of International Medicine Research.* 2007 Jan-Feb;35(1):84-90.

16. Kusum M, Klinbuayaem V, et al. Preliminary efficacy and safety of oral suspension SH, combination of five Chinese medicinal herbs, in people living with HIV/AIDS; the phase two study. *Journal of the Medical Association of Thailand.*

2004 Sep;87(9):1065-70.

17. Sangkitporn S, Shide L, et al. Efficacy and safety of Zidovudine and Zalcitabine combined with a combination of herbs in the treatment of HIV-infected Thai patients. *Southeast Asian Journal of Tropical Medicine*. 2005 May;36(3):704-708.

18. Wei X, Zhang J, et al. Astragalus mongholicus and Polygonum multiflorum's protective function against cyclophosphamide inhibitory effect on thymus. *American Journal of Chinese Medicine*. 2004;32(5):669-80.

Chapter 5 - Anemia and Leukopenia

1. Zheng KY, Choi RC, et al. Flavonoids from radix Astragali induce the expression of erythropoietin in cultured cells: a signaling mediated via the accumulation of hypoxia-inducible factor-1alpha. *Journal of Agricultural and Food Chemistry*. 2011 Mar 9;59(5):1697-1704.

2. Gao QT, Cheung JK, et al. A Chinese herbal decoction prepared from radix astragali and radix Angelicae sinensis induces the expression of erythropoietin in cultured Hep3B cells. *Planta Medica* 2008 Mar;74(4):392-5.

3. Zheng KY, Choi RC, et al. The expression of erythropoietin triggered by danggui buxue tang, a Chinese herbal decoction prepared from radix Astragali and radix Angelica sinensis, is mediated by the hypoxia-inducible factor in cultured HEK293T cells. *Journal of Ethnopharmacology*. 2010 Oct 28;132(1):259-67.

4. Zhu X, Zhu B. Effect of Astragalus membranaceus injection on megakaryocyte hematopoiesis in anemic mice. *Hua Xi Yi Ke Da Xue Xue Bao (Journal of West China University of Medical Sciences)*. 2001 Dec;32(4):590-2.

5. Huang WM, Qian XH, Zhao DH. Astragalus polysaccharides-induced gamma-globulin mRNA expression in K562 cells. *Nan Fang Yi Ke Da Xue Bao (Journal of Southern Medical University)*. 2009 May;29(5):939-42.

6. Shimizu N, Tomodo M, et al. An acidic polysaccharide having activity on the reticuloendothelial system from the root of Astragalus mongholicus. *Chemical and Pharmaceutical Bulletin (Tokyo)*. 1991 Nov;39(11):2969-72.

7. Lu Y, Feng X, Zhu B. Study on effect of Astragalus membranaceus injection on hematopoiesis in anemic mice with mylosuppression. *Zhong Yao Cai (Journal of Chinese Medicinal Materials)*. 2005 Sep;28(9):791-3.

8. Xue JX, Jiang Y, Yan YQ. Effects of the combination of Astragalus membranaceus (Fisch.)Bge. (AM), tail of Angelica sinensis (Oliv.) Diels. (TAS), Cyperus rotundus L. (CR), Liguisticum chuanxiong Hort. (LC) and

Peonia veitchii Lynch (PV) on the hemorrheological changes in normal rats. *Zhongguo Zhong Yao Za Zhi (China Journal of Chinese Materia Medica)*. 1993 Oct;18(10):621-3, 640.

9. Chang MS, Kim do R, et al. Treatment with Astragali raxix and Angelica radix enhances erythropoietin gene expresson in the cyclophosphamide-induced anemic rat. *Journal of Medical Food*. 2009 June;12(3):637-42.

10. Yang M, Chan GC, et al. An herbal decoction of Radix astragali and Radix angelica sinensis promotes hematopoiesis and thrombopoiesis. *Journal of Ethnopharmacology*. 2009 July 6;124(1):87-97.

11. Dong TT, et al. Chemical and biological assessment of a Chinese herbal decoction containing radix Astragali and radix Angelicae sinensis:Determination of drug ratio in having optimized properties. *Journal of Agricultural and Food Chemistry*. 2006 Apr5;54(7):2767-74.

12. Lei Y, Wang JH, Chen KJ. Comparative study on angiogenesis effect of Astragalus membranaceus and Angelica sinensis in chick embryo choriollantoic membrane. *Zhongguo Zhong Yao Za Zhi (China Journal of Chinese Materia Medica)*. 2003 Sept;28(9):876-8.

13. Gao Q, Li J, et al. Verification of the formulation and efficacy of Danggui Buxue Tang (a decoction of Radix Astragali and Radix Sinensis): an exemplifying systemic approach to revealing the complexity of Chinese herbal medicine formulae. *Chinese Medicine*. 2007 Nov:12.

14. Zhan JY, Zheng KY, et al. Chemical and biological assessment of Angelica Sinenesis Radix after processing with wine: and orthogonal array design to reveal the optimized conditions. *Journal of Agriculture and Food Chemistry*. 2012 June 8;59(11):6091-98.

15. Zheng KY, Coi RC, et al. The membrane permeability of Astragali radix derived formononetin and calycosin is increased by Angelica sinenis radix in Caco-2 cells: a synergistic action of an ancient herbal decoction danggui buxue tang. *Journal of Pharmaceutical and Biomedical Analysis*. 2012 May 31.

16. Huang GC, Wu LS, et al. Immuno-enhancement effects of Huang Qi Liu Yi Tang in a murine model of cyclophosphamide-induced leucopenia. *Journal of Ethnopharmacology*. 2007 Jan 19;109(2):229-35.

17. Yang BH, Zhu LQ, et al. Effects of Astragalus membranaeus and Panax notoginseng on the transformation of bone marrow stem cells and proliferation of EPC in vitro. *Zhonguo Zhong Yao Za Zhi (China Journal of Chinese Materia Medica)* 2005 Nov;30(22):1761-3.

Chapter 6 - Cancer

1. Kelly BC, Ikonomu MG. Flesh residues concentrations of organochloride pesticides in farmed and wild salmon from British Columbia, Canada. *Environmental Toxicology and Chemistry.* 2011 Nov;30(11):2456-64.

2. Vakonaki E, Androutsopoulos VP, et al. Pesticides and oncogenic modulation. *Toxicology* 2013 May 10;307:42-5.

3. Hermanowicz A, Nawarska Z, et al. The neutrophil function and infectious diseases in workers occupationally exposed to organochloride insecticides. *International Archives of Environmental Health.* 1982;50(4):329-40.

4. Falck F, Ricci A, Wolff MS. Pesticides and polychlorinated biphenyl residues in human breast lipids and their relation to breast cancer. *Journal of the National Cancer Institute* 1992;47:143-146.

5. Weir D, Shapiro M. *Circle of Poison; Pesticides and People in a Hungry World.* 1981. University of California Press.

6. Waldbott GL. Organophosphates. *Health effects of Environmental Pollutants.*1978:232-234. CV Mosely.

7. Li Y, Liu X, Xue SZ. Antidotal effect of glucoside extracted from astragalus membranaceus on dimethoate intoxication in guinea pigs. *La Medicina del Lavoro (Journal of Labor Medicine).*1998;89 Suppl 2:S136-41.

8. Morgan DP. Organophosphate cholinesterase-inhibiting pesticides. *Recognition and Management of Pesticide Poisonings, 2nd edition.* U.S. Environmental Protection Agency. Office of Pesticide Programs.1977:4-8.

9. Chatfield KB. Treatment of pesticide poisoning with acupuncture. *American Journal of Acupuncture.* 1985 Dec; 13:339-345.

10. Karagueuzian HS, White C, et al. Cigarette smoke radioactivity and lung cancer risk. *Nicotine and Tobacco Research.* 2012 Jan;14(1):79-90.

11. Palupi E, Jayanegara A, Ploeger A, Kahl J. Comparison of nutritional quality between conventional and organic dairy products: a meta-analysis. *Journal of the Science of Food and Agriculture.* 2012. Nov;(14): 2774-81.

12. Hunter D, Foster M, et al. Evaluation of the micronutrient composition of plant foods produced by organic and conventional agricultural methods. *Critical Reviews of Food, Science, and Nutrition.* 2011 July;(6):571-82.

13. Roberts JR, Karr CJ. Pesticide exposure in children. *Pediatrics.* 2012 Dec;130(6):e1765-88.

14. Zhang ZX, Qi F, et al. Effect of 5-fluorouracil in combinaton with Astragalus membranaccus on amino acid metabolism in mice model of gastric carcinoma. *Zhonghua Wei Chang Wai Ke Za Zhi (Chinese Journal of Integrated Traditional and Western Medicine)*. 2006 Sept;9(5):445-447.

15. Wei WY, Wu K, Wang XT. Effects of 5-FU combined compound ginseng and astragalus on biological behavior of human gastric cancer MGC-803 cells. *Zhongguo Zhong Xi Yi Jie He Za Zhi (Chinese Journal of Integrated Traditional and Western Medicine)*.2012 Dec;32(12):1647-51.

16. Liu HL, Chen XY, et al. The synergistic and toxicity-reducing effects of zhengqifuzheng injection on mice with 60Co radiotherapy. *Zhong Yao Cai (Journal of Chinese Materia Medica)*. 2009 Nov;32(11):1711-15.

17. Li K, Kuang WJ, et al. Anti-tumor effects of Astragalus on hepatocellular carcinoma in vivo. *Indian Journal of Pharmacology* 2012 Jan;44(1):78-81.

18. Cui R, He J, et al. Suppressive effect of Astragalus membranaceus (Bunge) on chemical hepatocarcinogenesis in rats. *Cancer Chemotherapy and Pharmacology.* 2003 Jan;51(1): 75-80.

19. Tian QE, De Li H, et al. Effects of Astragalus polysaccharides on P-glycoprotein efflux pump function and protein expression in H22 hepatoma cells in vitro. *BMC Complementary and Alternative Medicine.* 2012 July 11;12:94. Doi: 10.1186/1472-6882-12-94.

20. Huang C, Xu D, et al. Reversal of P-glycoprotein-mediated multidrug resistance of human hepatic cancer cells by Astragaloside II. *Journal of Pharmacy and Pharmacology.* 2012 Dec;64(12):1741-50.

21. Jia Y, Zuo D, et al. Astragaloside IV inhibits doxonubicin-induced cardionyocyte apoptosis mediated by mitochondrial apoptotic pathway via activating the P13K/Akt pathway. *Chemical and Pharmaceutical Bulletin.* 2014;62(1):45-53.

22. Ye MN, Chen HF, et al. Effects of astragalus polysaccharide on proliferation and Akt phosphorylation of the basal-like breast cancer cell line. Zhong Xi Jie He Xue Bao *(Journal of Chinese Integrative Medicine)*. 2011 Dec;9(12):1339-46.

23. Auyeung KK, Law PC, Ko JK. Astragalus saponins induce apoptosis via an ERK-independent NF-kappaB signaling pathway in the human hepatocellular HepG2 cell line. *International Journal of Molecular Medicine.* 2009 Feb;23(2):189-96.

24. Chu DT, Lepe-Zuniga J, et al. Fractionated extract of Astragalus membranaceus, a Chinese medicinal herb, potentiates LAK cell cytotoxicity generated by a low dose of recombinant interleukin-2. *Journal of Clinical and*

Laboratory Immunology 1988 Aug;26(4): 183-7.

25. Wang Y, Qian XJ, et al. Phytochemicals potentiate interleukin-2 generated lymphokine-activated killer cell cytotoxicity against murine renal cell carcinoma. *Molecular Biotherapy* 1992 Sep;4(3): 143-6.

26. Nalbantsoy A, Nesil T, et al. Evaluation of the immunomodulatory properties in mice and in vitro anti-inflammatory activity of cycloartane type saponins from Astragalus species. *Journal of Ethnopharmacology* 2012 Jan 31;139(2):574-581.

27. Dong JC, Dong XH. Comparative study on effect of Astragalus injection and interleukin-2 in enhancing anti-tumor metastasis action of dendrite cells. *Zhongguo Zhong Xi Yi Jie He Za Zhi (Chinese Journal of Traditional and Chinese Medicine)*. 2005 Mar;25(3):236-9.

28. Guo L, Bai SP. Astragalus polysaccharide injection integrated with vinorelbine and cisplatin for patients with advanced non-small cell lung cancer: effects on quality of life and survival. *Medical Oncology*. 2011 Sep 18.(Epub)

29. Chen HW, Lin IH, et al. A novel infusible botanically-derived drug, PG2, for cancer-related fatigue: a phase II double-blind, randomized placebo-controlled study. *Clinical Investigations in Medicine*. 2012 Feb 1;35(1):E1

30. Lee JJ, Lee JJ. A phase II study of an herbal decoction that includes Astragalus radix for cancer-associated anorexia in patients with advanced cancer. *Integrated Cancer Therapies*. 2010 Mar;9(1):24-31.

31. Dong J, Gu HL. Effects of large dose of Astragalus membranaceus on the dendritic cell induction of peripheral mononuclear cell and antigen presenting ability to dendritic cells in children with leukemia. *Zhongguo Zhong Xi Yi Jie He Za Zhi (Chinese Journal of Traditional and Chinese Medicine)*. 2005 Oct;24(10): 872-875.

32. Shao P, Zhao LH, et al. Regulation and function of dendritic cells by Astragalus mongholicus polysaccharides. *International Immunopharmacology*. 2006 Jul;6(7):1161-6.

33. Liu QY, Yao YM, et al. Astragalus polysaccharides regulate T cell-mediated immunity via CD11c(high)CD45RB(low) DCs in vitro. *Journal of Ethnopharmacology*. 2011 July 14;136(3):457-64.

34. Zhang D, Zhuang Y, et al. Investigation of effects and mechanisms of total flavonoids of Astragalus and calycosin on human erythroleukemia cells. *Oxidative Medicine and Cellular Longevity*. 2012;2012:209843.

35. Zhang D, Wang D, Yu Y. Effects and mechanisms of total flavonoids of

human astragalus radix and calycosis on inhibiting human erythroleukemia cell line K562. *Zhong Yao Za Zhi Zhongguo (Chinese Journal of Chinese Materia Medica).* 2011 Dec;36(24):3502-5.

36. Frokiaer H, Henningsen L, et al. Astragalus root and elderberry fruit extracts enhance the INF-Beta stimulatory effects of Lactobaccilus acidophilus in murine-derived dendritic cells. *PLoS One (Public Library of Science One).* 2012;7(10):e47878.

37. Zhang WJ, Hufnagl P, et al. Antiinflammatory activity of astragaloside IV is mediated by inhibition of NF-kappaB activation and adhesion molecule expression. *Thrombosis and Haemostasis* 2003 Nov;90(5):904-14.

38. Auyeung KK, Law PC, Ko JK. Novel anti-angiogenic effects of formononetin in human colon cancer cells and tumor xenograph. *Oncology Reports.* 2012 Dec;28(6):2188-94.

39. Auyeung KK, Woo PK, et al. Astragalus saponins modulate cell invasiveness and angiogenesis in human gastric adenocarcinoma cells. *Journal of Ethnopharmacology.* 2011 Aug 12.(Epub).

40. Li J, Bao Y, et al. Immunoregulatory and anti-tumor effects of polysaccharopeptide and Astragalus polysaccharides on tumor bearing mice. *Immunopharmacology and Immunotoxicology.* 2008;30(4):771-82.

41. Chu D, Sun Y, et al. F3, a fractionated extract of Astragalus membranaceus, potentiates lymphokine-activated killer cell cytotoxicity generated by low-dose recombinant interleukin-2. *Zhong Xi Yi Jie He Za Zhi (Chinese Journal of Traditional and Chinese Medicine).* 1990 Jan;10(1):34-6.

42. Zhao KW, Kong HY. Effect of Astragalan on secretion of tumor necrosis factors in human peripheral blood mononuclear cells. *Zhongguo Zhong Xi Yi Jie He Za Zhi (Chinese Journal of Traditional and Chinese Medicine).* 1993 May;13(5):263-5,259.

43. Kurashige S, Akuzawa Y, Endo F. Effects of astragali radix extract on carcinogenesis, cytokine production, and cytotoxicity in mice treated with a carcinogen, N-butyl-N'-butanolnitrosoamine. *Cancer Investigations.* 1999 ;17(1):30-35.

44. Wang JY, Ma GW, et al. Effect of cellular immune supportive treatment on immunity of esophageal carcinoma patients after modern two-field lymph node dissection. *Ai Zheng.* 2007 July;26(7): 778-81.

45. Wang J, Ito H, Shimura K. Enhancing effect of antitumor polysaccharide from Astragalus or Radix hedysarum on C3 cleavage production of macrophages in

mice. *Japanese Journal of Pharmacology* .1989 Nov;51(3):432-4.

46. Zhao TH. Positive modulation action of shengmaisan with astragalus membranaceus on anti-tumor activity of LAK cells. *Zhongguo Zhong Xi Yi Jie He Za Zhi (Chinese Journal of Traditional and Chinese Medicine)*. 1993 Aug;13(8):471-2, 453.

47. Cho WC, Leung KN. In vitro and in vivo anti-tumor effects of Astragalus membranaceus. *Cancer Letters*. 2007 July8;252(1):43-54.

48. Na D, Liu FN, et al. Astragalus extract inhibits destruction of gastric cancer cells to mesothelial cells by anti-apoptosis. *World Journal of Gastroenterology*. 2009 Feb 7;15(5):570-7.

49. Rittenhouse JR, Lui PD, Lau BH. Chinese medicinal herbs reverse macrophage suppression induced by urological tumors. *Journal of Urology*. 1991 Aug;146(2):486-90.

50. Li Q, Bao JM, et al. Inhibiting effect of Astragalus polysaccharides on the functions of CD4+CD25 high Treg cells in the tumor microenvironment of human hepatocellular carcinoma. *Chinese Medical Journal (Engl)*. 2012 Mar;125(5):786-93.

51. Jiang J, Wojnowski R, et al. Suppression of proliferation and invasive behavior of human metastatic breast cancer cells by dietary supplement BreastDefend. *Integrative Cancer Therapies*. 2011. June;10(2):192-200.

52. Jiang J, Thyagarajan-Sahu A, et al. BreastDefend prevents breast to lung cancer metastases in an orthotopic animal model of triple-negative human breast cancer. *Oncology Reports*. 2012 Oct;28(4):1139-45.

53. Frenkel M, Abrams DI, et al. Integrating dietary supplements into cancer care. *Integrative Cancer Therapy*. 2013 Feb 25.

Chapter 7- Heart Disease
1. Chen XJ, Meng D, etal. Protective effect of astragalosides on myocardial injury by isoproterenol in SD rats. *American Journal of Chinese Medicine*. 2006;34(6):1015-25.

2. Zhang WD, Chen H, et al. Astragaloside IV from Astragalus membranaceus shows cardioprotection during myocardial ischemia in vivo and vitro. *Planta Medica*. 2006 Jan;72(1):4-8.

3. Zhang W, Zhang C, et al. Quantitative determination of Astragaloside IV, a natural product with cardioprotective activity, in plasma, urine, and other

biological samples by HPLC coupled with tandem mass spectrometry. *Journal of Chromatography. B, Analytical Technologies in the Biomedical and Life Sciences.* 2005 Aug 5;822(1-2): 170-7.

4. Wu JH, Li Q, et al. Formononetin, an isoflavone, relaxes isolated aorta through endothelium-dependent and endothelium-independent pathways. *Journal of Nutritional Biochemistry.* 2010 July;21(7): 613-20.

5. Zhang WD, Zhang, C, et al. Astragaloside IV dilates aortic vessels from normal and spontaneously hypertensive rats through endothelium-dependent and endothelium-independent ways. *Planta Medica.* 2006 June;72(7):621-6

6. Jiang C, Gu X, et al. Influence of lypholized Radix Astragali powder injection on hemodynamics of dogs with myocardial ischemia. *Sheng Wu YI Xue Gong Cheng Xue Za Zhi (Journal of Biomedical Engineering).* 2010 Feb ;27(1): 74-9.

7. Chen LX, Liao JZ, Guo WQ. Effects of Astragalus membranaceus on left ventricular function and oxygen free radical in acute myocardial infarction patients and mechanism of its cardiotonic action. *Zhongguo Zhong Xi Yi Jie He Za Zhi (Journal of Integrated Traditional and Western Medicine).* 1995 Mar;15(3):141-3.

8. Ma X, Zhang K, et al. Extracts of Astragalus membranaceus limit myocardial cell death and improve cardiac function in a rat model of myocardial ischemia. *Journal of Ethnopharmacology.* 2013 Aug 19 pii:S0378-8741(13)00537-0.

9. You Y, Duan Y, et al. Anti-atherosclerotic function of astragali radix extract: downregulation of adhesion molecules in vitro and vivo. *BMC Complementary and Alternative Medicine.* 2012 Apr 26;2:54 doi; 10.1186/1472-6882-12-5

10. Li SQ, Yuan RX, Gao H. Clinical observation on the treatment of ischemic heart disease with Astragalus membranaceus. *Zhongguo Zhong Xi Yi Jie He Zhi (Journal of Integrated Traditional and Western Medicine).* 1995 Feb;15(2):77-80.

11. Ai P, Yong G, et al. Aqueous extract of Astragali Radix induces human natriuresis through enhancement of renal responce to atrial natriuretic peptide. *Journal of Ethnopharmacology.* 2008 Mar 28;116(3):413-21.

12. Rui T, Yang YZ, Zhou TS. Effects of Astragalus membranaceus on electrophysiological activities of acute experimental Coxsackie B3 myocarditis in mice. *Zhongguo Zhong Xi Yi Jie He Za Zhi (Journal of Integrated Traditional and Western Medicine).* 1994 May;14(5):392-4.

13. Peng TQ, Yang YZ, Zhou TS. Effects of Astragalus membranaceus on coxsacki B3 virus RNA in mice. *Zhongguo Zhong Xi yi Jie He Za Zhi (Journal of Integrated Traditional and Western Medicine).* 1994 Nov;14(11):664-6.

14. Guo Q, Peng TQ, Yang YZ. Effect of Astragalus membranaceus on Ca2+ influx and coxsackie virus B3 RNA replication in cultured neonatal rat heart cells. *Zhongguo Zhong Xi Yi Jie He Za Zhi (Journal of Integrated Traditional and Western Medicine).* 1995 Aug;15(8):483-5.

15. Peng T, Yang Y, et al. The inhibitory effect of Astragalus membranaceus on coxsackie B3 virus RNA replication. *Chinese Medical Society Journal.* 1995 Sep 10(3): 146-50.

16. Lu S, Zheng J, Yang D. Effects of Astragaloside in treating myocardial Sarco/ Endoplasmic C(2+)-ATPase of viral myocarditis mice. *Zhongguo Zhong Xi Yi Jie He Za Zhi (Journal of Integrated Traditional and Western Medicine).* 1999 Nov;19(11) 672-4.

17. Xiong D, Yang Y, Su Y. Experimental study on treatment of viral myocarditis in mice by integrated Chinese and western medicine. *Zhongguo Zhong Xi Yi Jie He Za Zhi. (Journal of Integrated Traditional and Western Medicine).* 1998 Aug;18(8):480-2.

18. Gu W, Yang YZ, He MX. A study on combination therapy of western and traditional Chinese medicine of acute viral myocarditis. *Zhongguo Zhong Xi Yi Jie He Za Zhi. (Journal of Integrated Traditional and Western Medicine).* 1996 Dec; 16(12):713-6.

19. Zhang ZC, Li SJ, et al. Effect of astragaloside on cardiomyocyte apoptosis in murine coxsackie virus B3 myocarditis. *Journal of Asian Natural Product Research.* 2007 Mar;9(2):145-51.

21. Guo Q, Peng TQ, Yang YZ. Effect of Astragalus membranaceus on Ca2+ influx and coxsackie virus B3 RNA replication in cultured neonatal rat heart cells. *Zhonguo Zhong Xi Yi Jie He Za Zhi. (Journal of Integrated Traditional and Western Medicine).* 1995 Aug;15(6):483-5.

21. Chen XJ, Bian ZP, et al. Cardiac protective effect of Astragalus on viral myocarditis mice: comparison with Perindopril. *American Journal of Chinese Medicine.* 2005;34(3) 493-502.

22. Yuan WL, Chen HZ, Zhou TS. Effect of Astragalus membranaceus on electrical activities of coxsackie B-2 virus-infected rat myocardial cells in culture. *Zhong Xi Yi Jie He Za Zhi (Chinese Journal of Modern Developments in Traditional Medicine).* 1989 June;9(6):355-7.

23. Yuan WL, Chen HZ, et al. Effect of Astragalus membranaceus on electrical activities of cultured rat beating heart cells infected with Coxsackie B-2 virus. *Chinese Medical Journal (Engl).* 1990 Mar;103(3):177-82.

24. Yang YZ, Jin PY, et al. Treatment of experimental Coxsackie B-3 viral myocarditis with Astragalus membranaceus in mice. *Chinese Medical Journal (Engl).* 1990 Jan;103(1):14-18.

25. Rui T, Yang Y, et al. Effect of Astragalus membranaceus on electrophysiological activities of acute experimental Coxsackie B-3 viral myocarditis in mice. *Chinese Medical Sciences Journal.* 1993 Dec;8(4):203-6.

26. Ye G, Tang Yh, et al. Characterization of anti-Coxsackie virus B3 constituents of radix Astragali by high-performance liquid chromatography coupled with electrospray ionization tandem mass spectrometry. *Biomedical Chromatography.* 2010 Nov;24(11):1147-51.

27. Zhao J, Yang P, et al. Therapeutic effects of astragaloside IV on myocardial injuries: Mult-target identification and network analysis. *PLoS One (Public Library of Science One).* 2012;7(9):e44938. Epub Sept 17.

28. Zhang JG, Yang N, He H. Effect of astragalus injections on serum apoptosis relevant factors in patients with chronic heart failure. *Zhong Xi Yi Jie He Za Zhi (Chinese Journal of Integrated Traditional and Western Medicine* 2005 May;25(5):400-3.

29. Luo HM, Dai RH, Li Y. Nuclear cardiology study on effective ingredients of Astragalus membranaceus in treating heart failure. *Zhongguo Zhong Xi Yi Jie He Za Zhi (Chinese Journal of Integrated Traditional and Western Medicine).* 1995 Dec;15(12):707-9.

30. Ma J, Peng A, Lin S. Mechanisms of the therapeutic effect of Astragalus membranaceus on sodium and water retention in experimental heart failure. *Chinese Medical Journal (Engl).* 1998 Jan;111(1):17-23.

31. Ma L, Guan ZZ. Effect of Astragalus injection on left ventricular remodeling and apoptotic gene caspase-3 in rats after myocardial infarction. *Zhongguo Zhong Xi Yi Jie He Za Zhi (Chinese Journal of Integrated Traditional and Western Medicine).* 2005 July;25(7):645-9.

32. Xu XL, Ji H, et al. Cardioprotective effects of Astragali radix against isoproterenol-induced myocardial injury in rats and its possible mechanism. *Phytotherapy Research* 2008 Mar;22(3):389-94.

33. Xu XL, Chen XJ, et al. Astragaloside IV improved intracellular calcium handling in hypoxia-reoxygenated cardiomyocytes via the sarcoplasmic reticulum Ca-ATPase. *Pharmacology.* 2008;81(4):325-32.

34. Zhou JY, Fan Y, et al. Effects of components isolated from Astragalus membranaceus(Bunge.) on cardiac function injured by myocardial ischemia

reperfusion in rats. *Zhongguo Zhong Yao Za Zhi (Chinese Journal of Chinese Materia Medica)*. 2000 May;25(5) 300-2.

35. Chen JX, Wang SR, et al. Effect of different drug dosage to activate blood circulation and to nourish qi on cardiac function and structure of congestive heart failure rats after acute myocardial infarction. *Zhongguo Zhong Yao Za Zhi (China Journal of Chinese Materia Medica)*. 2003 May;28(5):446-9.

36. Su D, Yan HR, et al. Effects of Astragalus membranaceus on cardiac function and SERCA2a gene expression in myocardial tissues of rats with chronic heart failure. *Zhong Yao Cai (Journal of Chinese Medicinal Materials)* 2009. Jan; 32(1):85-8.

37. Zhang WD, Zhang C, et al. Preclinical pharmacokinetics and tissue distribution of a natural cardioprotective agent astragaloside IV in rats and dogs. *Life Sciences*. 2006 July 17;(8):808-15.

38. Fu S, Zhang J, et al. Huangqi injection (a traditional Chinese patent medicine) for chronic heart failure: a systemic review. *(PLoS One Public Library of Science One)*. 2011May 6;6(5):e 19604. Doi:10.1371/journal.pone.0019604.

39. de Longeril M, Salen P, et al. Cholesterol lowering, cardiovascular diseases, and the rosuvastatin-JUPITER controversy:a critical reappraisal. *Archives of Internal Medicine*. 2010 June 28;170(12):1032-6.

40. Cheng Y, Tang K, et al. Astragalus polysaccharides lowers plasma cholesterol through mechanisms distinct from statins. *PLos One (Public Library of Science One)*. 2011;6(11):e27437.

41. Wang D, Zhuang Y, et al. Study on the effects of total flavonoids of Astragalus on atherosclerosis formation and potential mechanisms. *Oxidative Medicine and Cellular Longevity.* 2012:2012:282383. Epub 2012 Jan 29.

42. You Y, Duan Y, et al. Anti-atherosclerotic function of Astragali radix: downregulation of adhesion molecules. *BMC Complementary and Alternative Medicine*. 2012 Apr 26;12(1):54.

43. Zhao J, Zhu H, et al. Naoxintong protects against atherosclerosis through lipid-lowering and inhibiting maturation of dendritic cells in LDL receptor knockout mice fed a high-fat diet. *Current Pharmaceutical Design*. 2013;19(33):5891-6.

44. Kaiser C. Higher LDL level linked to lower incidence of Afib. *Medical Page Today*. 2012 Jan12.

45. Lopez F, Agarwal SK, et al. Blood lipid levels, lowering medications, and the incidence of atrial fibrillation: The atherosclerosis risk in communities (ARIC)

study. *Circulation Arrhythmia and Electrophysiology.* 2012 Feb;5(1):155-62.

46. Schatz IJ, Masaki K, et al. Cholesterol and all-cause mortality in elderly people from the Honolulu Heart Program: a cohort study. *The Lancet.* 2001 Aug 4;358(9279):351-5.

47. Schupf N, Costa R, et al. Relationship between plasma lipids and all-cause mortality in nondemented elderly. *Journal of the American Geriatric Society.* 2005 Feb;53(2):219-26.

48. Kastelein JJ, Akdim F, et al. Simvastatin with or without ezetimibe in familial hypercholesterolemia. *New England Journal of Medicine* 2008 Apr 3:358(14):1431-43.

Chapter 8 - Brain and Nervous System

1. Luo Y, Qin Z, et al. Astragaloside IV protects against ischemia brain injury in a murine model of transient focal ischemia. *Neuroscience Letters.* 2004 June 17;363(3):218-23.

2. Qu YZ, Li M, et al. Astragaloside IV attenuates cerebral ischemia-reperfusion-induced increase in permeability of the blood-brain barrier in rats. *European Journal of Pharmacology.* 2009 Mar;16:606(1-3):137-41.

3. Chen CC, Lee HC, et al. Chinese herb astragalus membranaceus enhances recovery of hemorrhagic stroke: Double blind, placebo controlled, randomized study. *Evidence Based Complementary and Alternative Medicine.* 2012;2012:708452. Epub 2012 Mar 12.

4. Fang WK, Ko FY, et al. The proliferation and migration effects of huangqi on RSC96 Schwann cells. *American Journal of Chinese Medicine.* 2009;37(5):945-59.

5. Zhu L, Shi ZY, et al. Prevention of Rhodiola-Astragalus membranaceus compounds against simulated plateau hypoxia brain injury in rat. *Space Medicine and Medical Engineering (Beijing).* 2005 Aug;18(4): 303-5.

6. He X, Li C, Yu S. Protective effects of radix Astragali against anoxic damages to in vitro cultured neurons. *Journal of Tongji Medical University.* 2000;29(2): 136-7.

7. Hong GX, Qin WC, Huang LS. Memory improving effect of Astragalus membranaceus. *Zhonguo Zhong Yao Za Zhi (China Journal of Chinese Materia Medica).* 1994 Nov;19(11):687-8, 704.

8. Deitrich R, Zimatkin S, Pronko . Oxidation of ethanol in the brain and its consequences. *Alcohol Research and Health.* 2006 29(4):266-273.

9. Zacharis S. Overwiew: How is alcohol metabolized by the body. *Alcohol Research and Health.* 2006 29(4):245-254.

10. Yu DH, Bao YM, et al. Protection of PC12 cells against superoxide-induced damage, by isoflavonoids from Astragalus mongholicus. *Biomedical and Environment Sciences.* 2009 Feb;22(1):50-4.

11. Forsynth CB, Shannon KM, et al. Increased intestinal permeability correlates with sigmoid mucosa alpha-synuclein staining and endotoxin exposure markers in early Parkinson's disease. *PLoS (Public Library of Science)* 2011;6(12):e28032. Doi;10.1371/journal.pone 0028032.Epub 2011 Dec 1.

12. Chan WS, Durairajan SS, et al. Neuroprotective effects of Astragaloside IV in 6-hydroxydopamine-treated primary nigral cell culture. *Neurochemistry International.* 2009 Nov;55(6):414-22.

13. Zhang ZG, Wy L, et al. Astragaloside IV prevents MPP(+)-induced SH-SY5Y cell death via the inhibition of Bax-mediated pathways and ROS production. *Molecular and Cellular Biochemistry.* 2012 May;364(1-2):209-16.

14. Tohda C, Tamura T, et al. Promotion of axonal maturation and prevention of memory loss in mice by extracts of Astragalus mongholicus. *British Journal of Pharmacology.* 2006 Nov;14(5):532-41.

15. Jia RZ, Jiang L, et al. Neuroprotective effects of Astragalus membranaceus on hypoxia-ischemia brain damage in neonatal rat hippocampus. *Zhongguo Zhong Yao Za Zhi (China Journal of Chinese Materia Medica).* 2003 Dec;28(12):1174-7.

16. Li WZ, Li WP, et al. Protective effect of extract of Astragalus on learning and memory impairments and neurons' apoptosis induced by glucocorticoids in 12-month-old male mice. *Anatomical Record.* 2011 June;294(6):1003-14.

17. Li WZ, Wu WY, et al. Protective effects of astragalosides on dexamethasone and Amyloid beta 25-35 induced learning and memory impairments due to decrease amyloid precursor protein expression in 12-month male rats. *Food and Chemical Toxicology.* 2012. June;50(6):1883-90.

18. Aldarmaa J, Liu Z, et al. Anti-convulsant effect and mechanism of Astragalus mongholicus extract in vitro and vivo: protection against oxidative damage and mitochondrial dysfunction. *Neurochemistry Research.* 2010 Jan;35(1):33-41.

19. Jalsrai A, Grecksch G, Becker A. Evaluation of the effects of Astragalus mongholicus saponin extract on central nervous system functions. *Journal of Ethnopharmacology.* 2010 Oct5:131(3);544-9.

20. Kim C, Ha H, et al. Induction of growth hormone by the roots of Astragalus

membranaceus in pituitary cell culture. *Archives of Pharmaceutical Research.* 2003 Jan;26(1):34-9.

Chapter 9 - Liver

1. Zhang ZL, Wen QZ, Liu CX. Hepatoprotective effects of Astragalus root. *Journal of Ethnopharmacology.* 1990 Sep;30(2):145-9.

2. Yan F, Zhang QY, et al. Synergistic hepatoprotective effect of Schizandrae ligans with Astragalus polysaccharides on chronic liver injury in rats. *Phytomedicine.* 2009 Sep;16(9):805-13.

3. Xiang KM, Chen XD. Effects of astragalosides on the induction of colorectal aberrant crypt foci by dimethylhydrazine and metabolizing enzymes in liver microsomes in rats. *Nan Fang Yi Ke Da Zue Bao (Journal of Southern Medical University).* 2010 July;30(7):1720-1, 1723.

4. Kwon HJ, Hyun SH, Choung SY. Traditional Chinese medicine improves dysfunction of peroxisome proliferators-activiated receptor alpha and microsomal triglyceride transfer protein on abnormalities in lipid metabolism in ethanol-fed rats. *Biofactors.* 2005;23(3);163-76.

5. Jia R, Cao L, et al. In vitro and in vivo hepatoprotective and antioxidant effects of Astragalus polysaccharides against carbon tetrachloride-induced hepatocyte damage in common carp (Cyprinus carpio). *Fish Physiology and Biochemistry.* 2011 Nov17.

6. Sun WY, Wei W, et al. Protective effect of extract from Paeonia lactiflora and Astragalus membranaceus against liver injury induced by bacillus Calmette-Guerin and lipopolysaccharide in mice. *Basic Clinical and Pharmacological Toxicology.* 2008 Aug;103(2):143-9.

7. Li X, Wang X, et al. Astragaloside IV suppresses collagen production of activated HSCs via oxidative stress-mediated p38 MAPK pathway. *Free Radicals in Biological Medicine.* 2013. Feb 28 pii: S0891-5849(13)00091-9.

8. Tan YW, Yin YM, Yu XJ. Influence of Salvia miltiorrhizae and Astragalus membranaceus on hemodynamics and liver fibrosis indexes in liver cirrhotic patients with portal hypertension. *Zhongguo Zhong Xi Yi Jie He Za Zhi (Chinese Journal of Integrated Traditional and Western Medicine).* 2001 May;21(5):351-3.

9. Yuan Y, Sun M, Li KS. Astragalus mongholicus polysaccharide inhibits lipopolysaccharide-induced production of TNF-alpha and interleukin-8. *World Journal of Gastroenterology.* 2009 Aug 7;15(29):3676-80.

10. Zhou X, Dai LL, et al. Study on the inhibitive effect if Astragalus injection

solution on hepatic fibrosis in rats. *Zhonghua Gan Zang Bing Za Zhi (Chinese Journal of Hepatology).* 2005 Aug;13(8):575-8.

11. Wang P, Liang YZ. Chemical composition and inhibitory effect on hepatic fibrosis of Danggui Buxue Decoction. *Filoterapia.* 2010 Oct;81(7):793-8.

12. Tong X, Chen GF, Lu Y. Uniform designed research on the active ingredients assembling of huangqi decoction for inhibition of DMN-induced liver fibrosis. *Zhongguo Zhong Xi Jie He Za Zhi (Chinese Journal of Integrated Traditional and Western Medicine).* 2011 Oct;31(10):1389-93.

13. Li X, Peng XD, et al. Inhibiting effects of denshensu, baical, astragalus, and Panax notoginseng saponins on hepatic fibrosis and their possible mechanisms. *Zhonghua Gan Zang Bing Za Zhi (Chinese Journal of Hepatology).* 2008 Mar;16(3):193-7.

14. Yang Y, Yang S, et al. Compound Astragalus and Salvia miltorrhiza extract exerts anti-fibrosis by mediating TGF-beta/Smad signaling in myofibroblasts. *Journal of Ethnopharmacology.* 2008 July23;118(2):264-70.

15. Sun WY, Wei W, ey al. Effects and mechanisms of extract from Paeonia lactiflora and Astragalus membranaceus on liver fibrosis induced by carbon tetrachloride in rats. *Journal of Ethnopharmacology.* 2007 July 25;112(3): 514-23.

16. Wang JJ, Li J, et al. Preventive effects of a fractionated polysaccharide from a traditional Chinese herbal medical formula (Yu Ping Feng San) on carbon tetrachloride-induced hepatic fibrosis. *Journal of Pharmacy and Pharmacology.* 2010 July;62(7):935-42.

17. Wang LX, Han ZW.The effect of Astragalus polysaccharides on endotoxin-induced toxicity in mice. *Yao Xue Xue Bao (Acta Pharmaceutica Sinica).* 1992;27(1):5-9.

18. Wu L, Liu H, et al. Influence of a triplex superimposed treatment on HBV replication and mutation during treating chronic hepatitis B. *Zhonghua Shi Yan He Lin Chuang Bing Du Xue Za Zhi (Chinese Journal of Experimental and Clinical Virology)* 2001 Sep;15(3):236-8.

19. Wang S, Li J, et al. Anti-hepatitis B virus activities of astragaloside IV isolated from radix Astragali. *Biological and Pharmaceutical Bulletin.* 2009 Jan;32(1):132-5.

20. Du X, Zhao B, et al. Astragalus polysaccharides enhance immune responces of HBV DNA vaccination via promoting dendritic cell maturation and suppressing Treg frequency in mice. *International Immunopharmacology.* 2012 Dec;14(4):463-70.

21. Du X, Chen Y, et al. Astragalus polysaccharides enhance the humoral and cellular immune responces of hepatitis B surface antigen vaccination through inhibiting the expression of transforming growth factor beta and the frequency of regulatory T cells. *FEMS Immunology and Medical Microbiology*. 2011 Nov;63(2):228-35.

22. Chen Y, Wang D, et al. Astragalus polysaccharide and oxymatrine can synergistically improve the immune efficacy of Newcastle disease vaccine in chickens. *International Journal of Biological Macromolecules*. 2010 May 1;46(4):425-8.

Chapter 9 - Lupus

1. Zhao XZ. Effects of Astragalus membraceus and Tripterygium hypoglancum on natural killer cell activity of peripheral blood mononucleuar in systemic lupus erythematosus. *Zhongguo Zhong Xi Yi Jie He Za Zhi (Chinese Journal of Integrated Traditional and Western Medicine)* 1992 Nov;12(11):669-71, 645.

2. Su L, Mao JC, Gu JH. Effect of intravenous drip infusion of cyclophosphamide with high-dose Astragalus injection in treating lupus nephritis. *Zhong Xi Yi Jie He Xue Bao (Journal of Chinese Integrative Medicine)*. 2007 May;5(3):272-5.

3. Cai XY, Xu YL,Lin XJ. Effects of radix Astragali injection on apoptosis of lymphocytes and immune function in patients with systemic lupus erythematosis. *Zhonguo Zhong Xi Yi Jie He Za Zhi (Chinese Journal of Integrated Traditional and Western Medicine)*. 2006 May;26(5):443-5.

4. Wang H, Wang J, et al. A clinical study on leucopenia in patients with systemic lupus erythematosus treated with radix astragali injection. *Journal of Lanzhou University Medical Sciences*. 2007. 01.

5. Pan FH Fang XH, et al. Radix Astragali: a promising new treatment option for systemic lupus erythematosus. *Medical Hypothesis*. 2008 Aug;71(2):311-2.

Chapter 10 - Aging and Life Extension.

1. Li WZ, Li WP, Yin YY. Effects of AST and ASI on metabolism of free radical in senescent rats treated by HC. *Zhonguo Zhong Yao Za Zhi (China Journal of Chinese Maertia Medica)*. 2007 Dec;32(23):2539-42.

2. Yang B, Ji C, et al. Protective effect of astragaloside IV against matrix metalloproteinase-1 expression in ultraviolet irradiated human dermal fibroblasts. *Archives of Pharmaceutical Research*. 2011 Sep;34(9):1553-60.

3. Liu X, Min W. Protective effects of astragaloside against ultraviolet A-induced photoaging in human fibroblasts. *Zhong Xi Yi Jie He Xue Bao (Journal of Chinese*

Integrative Medicine). 2011 Mar;9(3):328-32.

4. Hong MJ, Ko EB, et al. Inhibitory effect of Astragalus membranaceus root on matrix metalloproteinase-1 collagenase expression and procollagen destruction in ultraviolet B-irradiated human dermal fibroblasts by suppressing nuclear factor kappa-B activity. *Journal of Pharmaceutical Pharmacology*. 2013 Jan;65(1): 142-8.

5. Xu P, Jin G, Shen X. Effect of radix Astragalus on the contents of collagen in the aorta and lung of old rats. *Zhonguo Zhong Yao Za Zhi (China Journal of Chinese Materia Medica)*. 1991 Jan;16(1):49-50, 65.

6. Wang P, Zhang Z, et al. HDTIC-1 and HDTIC-2, two compounds extracted from Astragali radix, delay replicative senescence of human diploid fibroblasts. *Mechanisms of Ageing and Development*. 2003 Dec;124(10-12):1025-34.

7. Wang P, Zhang ZY, et al. Two isomers of HDTIC isolated from Astragali radix decrease the expression of p16 in 2BS cells. *Chinese Medical Journal (Engl)*. 2008 Feb 5;121(3):231-5.

8. Wang P, Zhang Z, et al. The two isomers of HDTIC compounds from Astragali radix slow down telomere shortening rate via attenuated oxidative stress and increasing DNA repair ability in human fetal lung diploid fibroblast cells. *DNA and Cell Biology*. 2010 Jan;29(1):33-9.

9. Shi R, He L, et al. The regulatory action of radix Astragali on M-cholinergic receptor of the brain of senile rats. *Journal of Traditional Chinese Medicine*. 2001 Sep;21(3):232-5.

10. Li XT, Zhang YK, et al. Mitochondrial protection and anti-aging activity of Astragalus polysaccharides and their potential mechanism. *International Journal of Molecular Science*. 2012;13(2):1747-61.

11. de Jesus BB, Schneeberger K, et al. The telomerase activator TA-65 elongates short telomeres and increases health span of adult/old mice without increasing cancer incidence. *Aging cell*. 2011 Aug10(4):604-21.

12. Xu T, Xu Y, et al. Reprogramming murine telomerase rapidly inhibits the growth of mouse cancer cells in vitro and vivo. *Molecular Cancer Therapy*. 2010 Feb;9(2): 438-49.

13. Shawi M, Autexier C. Telomerase, senescence and ageing. *Mechanisms of Ageing and Developement* 2008 Jan-Feb;129(1-2):3-10.

14. Mendelson AR, Larrick JW. Ectopic expression of telomerase safely increases health span and life span. *Rejuvination Research*. 2012 Aug;15(4):435-8.

15. Molgora B, Bateman R, et al. Functional assessment of pharmacological telomerase activators in human T cells. *Cells.* 2013, 2(1), 56-66.

16. Wang P, Zhang Z, et al. The two isomers of HDTIC compounds from Astrgali Radix slow down telomere shortening rate via attenuating oxidative stress and increasing DNA repair ability in human fetal lung diploid fibroblast cells. *DNA Cell Biology.* 2010 Jan;29(1):29(1):33-9.

17. Zhang, Lin S, et al. Environmental and occupational exposure to chemicals and telomere length in human studies. *Occupational and Environmental Medicine.* 2013 June 17.

18. Wang Y, Zhu YQ, et al. The protective effect of Astragalus membraceus extraction on cryopreserved primary-cultured human fetal hepatocytes. *Zhong Yao Cai (Journal of Chinese Medicinal Materials)* 2007 Dec;30(12):1151-4.

19. Liang P, Li H. Effects of astragalus membranaceus injection on sperm abnormality in Cd-induced rats. *Zhonghua Nan Ke Xue (National Journal of Andrology).* 2004 Jan;10(1):42-5.

20. Liu J, Liang P, et al. Effects of several Chinese herbal aqueous extracts on human sperm motility in vitro. *Andrologia.* 2004 Apr;36(2):78-83.

21. Kim W, Kim SH, et al. Astragalus membranaeus ameliorates reproductive toxicity induced by cyclophosphamide in male mice. *Phytotherapy Research.* 2012 Sept;26(9):1418-21.

Chapter 11 - Healing Injuries

1. Sevimli-Gur C, Onbasilar I, et al. In vivo growth stimulatory and in vivo healing studies on cycloartane-type saponins of Astragalus genus. *Journal of Ethnopharmacology.* 2011 April 12;134(3):844-50.

2. Huh Je, Nam DW, et al. Formonenetin accelerates wound repair by the regulation of early growth response factor-1 transcription factor through the phosphorylation of the ERK and p38 MAPK pathways. *International Immunopharmacology.* 2011 Jan;11(1):46-54.

3. He S, Yang Y, et al. Compound Astragalus and Salvia miltorrhiza extract inhibits cell proliferation, invasion and collagen synthesis in keloid fibroblasts by mediating transforming growth factor-beta/Smad pathway. *British Journal of Dermatology.* 2011 Oct 3.1365-2133.

4. Chen X, Peng LH, et al. The healing and anti-scar effects of astragaloside IV on wound repair in vitro and in vivo. *Journal of Ethnopharmacology.* 2012 Feb 15;139(3):721-7.

5. Liu HJ, Wang XP, et al. The effect of icarin and astragaloside 1 on the proliferation and differentiation of bone marrow stromal cells. *Zhong Yao Cai (Journal of Chinese Medicinal Materials).* 2006 Oct;29(10):1062-5.

6. Xu CJ, Gao F, et al. Effects of Astragalus polysaccharides-chitosan/polylactic acid scaffolds and bone marrow stem cells on repairing supra-alveolar periodontal defects in dogs. *Zhong Nan Da Xue Bao Yi Xue Ban (Journal of Central South University, Medical Sciences).* 2006 Aug;31(4):512-7.

7. Yao C, Gao F, et al. Experimental research of Astragalus polysaccharides collagen sponge in enhancing angiogenesis and collagen synthesis. *Zhoguo Xia Fu Chong Jian Wai Ke Za Zhi (Chinese Journal of Reparative and Reconstructive Surgery).* 2011 Dec;25(12):1481-5.

8. Wegiel B, Persson JL. Effect of a novel botanical agent Drynol Cibotin on human osteoblast cells and implications of osteoporosis: promotion of cell growth, calcium uptake and collagen production. *Phytotherapy Research.* 2010 June;24 Suppl 2:S139-47.

9. Kim MY, Park Y, et al. The herbal formula HT042 induces longitudinal bone growth in adolescent female rats. *Journal of Medical Food.* 2010 Dec;13(6):1376-84.

10. Xu C, Xian X, Guo F. An experimental study on effect of astragalus polysaccharides on chitosan/polylactctic acid scaffolds for repairing alveolar bone defects in dogs. *Zhongguo Xiu Fu Chong Jian Wai Ke Za Zhi (Chinese Journal of Reparative and Reconstructive Surgery).* 2007 July;21(7):748-752.

11. Kong XH, Niu YB, et al. Astragaloside II induces osteogenic activities of osteoblasts through bone morphogenic protein-2/MAPK and Smad 1/5/8 pathways. *International Journal of Molecular Medicine.* 2012 June;29(6): 1090-8 doi: 10.3892/ijmm.2012.941 Epub 2012 Mar 15.

12. Xie QF, Xie JH, et al. Effect of a derived herbal recipe from an ancient Chinese formula Danggui Buxue Tang, on ovariectomized rats. *Journal of Ethnopharmacology.* 2012 Oct pii:S0378-8741(12)00649-6.

13. Kang SC, Kim HJ, Kim MH. Effects of Astragalus membranaceus with supplemental calcium on bone mineral densisty and bone metabolism in calcium-deficient ovariectomized rats. *Biological and Trace Elements Research.* 2013, Jan;151(1):68-74.

14. Zheng YZ, Choi RC, et al. Ligustilide suppresses the biological properties of Danggui Buxue Tang: a Chinese medicine herbal decoction composed of radix Astragali and radix Angelica sinensis. *Planta Medica.* 2010. March;76(5)439-43.

15. Xiong M, Lai H, et al. Astragaloside IV attenuates impulse noise-induced trauma in guinea pig. *Acta Otolaryntology.* 2011 Aug;131(8):809-16.

16. Xiong M, He Q, et al. Radix Astragali injection enhances recovery from acute acoustical trauma. *Acta Otolaryntology.* 2011 Oct;131(10):1069-73.

17. Lu MC, Yao CH, et al. Effect of Astragalus membranaceus in rats on peripheral nerve regeneration: in vitro and in vivo studies. *Journal of Trauma.* 2010 Feb;68(2):434-40.

18. McAteer JA, Evan AP. The acute and long-term adverse effects of shock wave lithotripsy. *Seminars in Nephrology* 2008 March;28(2): 200-213.

19. Li X, He DL, et al. The protective effects of three components isolated from Astragalus membranaceus on shock wave lithotripsy induced kidney injury in rabbit model. *Zhonghua Yi Xue Za Zhi .* 2005 Aug17;85(31):2201-6.

20. Yuan Y, Sun M, Li KS. Astragalus mongholicus polysaccharide inhibits lipopolysaccharide-induced production of TNF-alpha and interleukin-8. *World Journal of Gastroenterology.* 2009 Aug 7;15(29):3676-80.

Chapter 12 - Astragalus and Inflammatory Diseases

1. Choi SI, Heo TR, et al. Alleviation of osteoarthritis by calycosin-7-O-beta-D-glucopyranoside (CG) isolated from Astragali radix (AR) in rabbit osteoarthritis (OA) model. *Osteoarthritis Cartilage.* 2007 Sep;15(9):1086-92.

2. Jiang JB, Qiu JD, et al. Therapeutic effects of Astragalus polysaccharides on inflammation and synovial apoptosis in rats with adjuvant-induced arthritis. *International Journal of Rheumatic Diseases.* 2010 Oct;13(4):396-405.

3. Yang LH, Qiu JD. Effects of Astragalus heteropolysaccharides on erythrocyte immune adherence function of mice with adjuvant-induced arthritis. *Yao Xue Xue Bao (Acta Pharmaceutica Sinica).* 2009 Dec;44(12):1364-70.

4. Gu X, Jiang D, et al. Effects of astragaloside IV on eosinophil activation induced by house mites. *Molecular Medicine Reports* 2012Apr 12.

5. Du Q, Gu XY, et al. Effects of astragaloside IV on the expressions of transforming growth factor-beta1 and thymic stromal lymphopoietin in a murine model of asthma. *Zhongghua Yi Xue Za Zhi* 2011 Nov 29;91(44):3139-42.

6. Li CC, Ye LP, et al. Effect of Radix Astragali on signal transducer and activator of transcription activator-4 and its mRNA expression in a rat model of asthma. *Zhonghua Er Ke Za Zhi (Chinese Journal of Pediatrics).* 2007 Oct;45(10):727-31.

7. Yuan X, Sun S, et al. Effects of astragaloside IV on IFN-gamma level and prolonged airway dysfunction in a murine model of chronic asthma. *Planta Medica*. 2011 March;77(4):328-33.

8. Qu ZH, Yang ZC. Inhibition airway remodeling and transforming growth factor-beta1/Smad signaling pathway by astragalus extract in asthmatic mice. *International Journal of Molecular Medicine*. 2012. April;29(4):564-8.

9. Matkovic Z, Zivkovic V, et al. Efficacy and safety of Astragalus membranaceus in the treatment of patients with seasonal allergic rhinitis. *Phytotherapy Research*. 2010 Feb;24(2):175-81.

10. Kim JH, Kim MH, et al. Effects of topical application of astragalus membranaceus on allergic dermatitis. *Immunopharmacology and Immunotoxicology*. 2013 Feb:35(1):151-6.

11. Prieto JM, Recio MC, et al. Influence of traditional Chinese anti-inflammatory medicinal plants on leukocytes and platelet functions. *Journal of Pharmacy and Pharmacology*. 2003. Sep;5(9):1275-82

INDEX

Symbols

5-FU (flourourcil) 47, 48
5-lipoxygenase 93

A

acetylaldehyde dehydrogenase 69
acetylaldehydes 69
acupuncture 66
acute loud noise trauma 88
adenovirus. *See* viruses
adriamycin 48
AGEs 29
   kidney damage 28
agriculture grown oils (omega-6) 21
alcoholism 68
allergic rhinitis 92
allergies 14, 91
alpha particles 44
alterative 26
Alzheimer's Disease 71, 72
   aluminum 72
   variant called ALS-PDC 72
Ames mutagenic test 12
amyloid 71
anemias 15
angina pain 60
angiogenesis 26
aplastic anemia 40
apoptosis 49
appetite (anorexia) 52
arctic root (Rhodiola) 67
arthritis 91
asthma 91
astragalans 9
astragaloside II 87
astragaloside IV 29, 34, 47, 61, 71,
     77, 88
   pregnancy 34
   protecting heart cells 48
   ulcerative wound healing 30
astragalosides 9

astragaloside IV 9, 11
astragalus
   reduces ulcer scarring 29
astragalus-rhodiola 67
atherosclerosis 27, 28
ATP (adenosine triphosphate) 62, 82
atrial fibrillation 64
autoimmunity 18
   gluten 18
axons 67

B

beany flavor 11
blood-brain barrier 66
blood thinning 12
bone mineral density 87
bone regeneration 86
Bovine Serum Albumin(BSA) 18
brain cells 66, 67
brain injuries 14
brain tissue, stress hormones and
     amyloid deposits 72
BreastDefend 56
bronchitis 33, 97
Bu Fei Wan 96
Bu Zhong Yi Qi Wan 95

C

cadmium 85
calcium supplementation and
     astragalus 87
calycosin 10
Campbell, Thomas 18
cancer 14, 35
candidiasis, systemic 34
cardiac enzymes, decreased release
     of 59
cardiac mitochondria 60
cardiomyopathy 27
casein 17
Center For Disease Control 20, 31
cerebral vascular accidents.
     See strokes

chemotherapeutic drugs 47
chemotherapy 15
chlorine 80
cholesterol 61
   HDL cholesterol 63
   LDL cholesterol 63
   Oxidized cholesterol 62
   reduction 63
chronic heart failure, severe 61
chronic obstructive pulmonary
   disease (COPD) 97
cigarettes 44, 45
cirrhosis 15, 76
cirrhotic scarring 76
cirrhotic tissue 75, 76
cisplatin 48, 57
Coenzyme Q10 or CoQ10 62
colony-stimulating factors 24
common colds 97
concussions 66, 67
congestive heart failure 59, 61
Cornell China study 18
coxsackie. *See* viruses
CREM 85
cryptosporidium 35
cultivating astragalus 11
cycloastragenol 10, 83
cyclophosphamide (Cytoxan) 78
cyclophosphamide (Cytoxin) 37,
   40, 48
cyclosporine 34
cytokine 24
   IL-1beta 34
cytokine production, altering 25
cytokine storm 34
cytomegalovirus 34

D

dang gui (Angelica sinensis) 64, 87
   ligustilide 87
Dang Gui Bu Xue Tang 31, 39, 95
   best ratio 39
DDT 42

deathcap mushrooms (Amanita
   phalloides) 77
dendrites 67
dendritic cells 51, 52, 53
diabetes 14, 27
   accelerates heart disease 27
   error in metabolism 22
   vision 30
diabetes, latent autoimmune
   (LADA) 19
diabetes, Type 1 17
   antibodies 19
   cow's milk, early introduction 17
   sixth chromosome 17
   trigger 17
   viral infection 17
diabetes, Type 2 19
   five main causes 19
   non-insulin dependent diabetes
   mellitus (NIDDM) 19
dimethylsulfoxide (DMSO) 85
dopamine 70
DR-6 (death receptor 6) 73

E

ear ringing. *See* tinnitus
E. coli 54, 70, 76
eczema 93
electrocardiogram (EKG) studies 60
elk antler extract 40
endophytes
   bacterial 9
   fungal 13
endotoxins 70, 76
ENHANCE trial 64
environmental illness 15
eosinophils 92
epilepsy 73
Epimedium 87
EPO. *See* erythropoietin
erythropoietin 38
essential fatty acids 21
etoposide 48

F

failure to thrive syndrome 15
fatigue 23
    moderate to severe 52
fats 21
    hydrogenated 21
    partially hydrogenated 21
fatty streak 63
ferrulic acid 39
fertility rates 85
fever 34
    reducing pro-inflammatory fever responses 34
flavonoids 10
foam cells 64
foot ulcers, non-healing 29
formononetin 29, 55
fractures 14, 86
free radical chemicals 29

G

GABA (gamma amino butyrate) 18
GAD (glutamic acid decarboxylase 18
GFRe 23
ginseng 10
glomerular filtration rate estimate 23
glutathione peroxidase (GSH-Px) 69
glycation end products (AGEs) 28
gut brain, the 70

H

HDL cholesterol. *See* cholesterol
HDTIC 81, 84
hearing loss, noise-induced 87
heart disease 14, 23
hemorrhagic stroke, acute 66
hepatitis 15
Hepatitis B 77
    reducing viral levels 77
    vaccine 77
HER2 57
Herb Pharm 98

herpes simplex 1 34
he shou wu (Polygonum multiflorum/ Reynoutria multiflora) 37
hexanal 11
HIF. *See* hypoxia-inducible factor
high fructose corn syrup 20
hippocampus 72, 73
    damage by stress 72
    destruction 72
HIV 34, 36
HMG-CoA reductase 62
homeostatic functions 26
honey frying astragalus 8
Horizon Herb Company 11
Horizon Herb Seed Company 98
HRE. *See* hypoxia response element
Huang Qi He Shou Wu Wan 96
Huang Qi Liu Yi Tang 40
Human Immunodeficiency Virus (HIV). *See* HIV
hydrogen peroxides 32
hyperaccumulators of selenium 13
hypertension 26, 59, 76
hypotension 26
hypoxia 67
hypoxia-inducible factor 38
hypoxia response element 38

I

immune deficiencies 14, 23
immune function, poor 35
immune suppression, reverse 33
immunosuppressive drugs 33
infections 14, 32
    reduce 34
inflammation 15, 23
inflammatory 51
influenza 97
insulin dependent diabetes. *See* diabetes, Type 1
insulin resistance 30
interactions between synthetic drugs and astragalus 14

interferons 24
interleukin-2 (Il-2) 14, 50
interleukin-8 90
interleukin-12 (IL-12) 53
interleukins 24, 31
isoflavonoids 10
    0.5% of hydroxy-3-methoxy-
        isoflavone-7 10

J

JUPITER study 63

K

Kaptchuck, Ted 8
kidney damage 78
kidney damage, AGEs-induced 28
kidney disease 14
kidney disease, diabetes-caused 25
kidney function and repair, enhance
        25
kidney stones 89

L

Lactobacillus acidophilus 54, 77
latent autoimmune diabetes (LADA)
        19
LDL cholesterol. *See* cholesterol
leukemia 53
leukopenia, causes of 39
Lewis and Clark Expedition 13
licorice 10
Lithotripsy 89
liver 75
liver disease 15
locoism 13
locoweed 13
lung disease 14
lupus 35, 78
    lupus-caused infection 78
Lyme disease 13

M

Mayway Corporation 97
M-cholinergic receptors 82
MDRs. *See* multidrug-resistant pumps

mental and physical exhaustion 15
mesangial cell 28
milk thistle (Silymarin marianis) 77
minerals 10
mitochondria 82
MMP 55
MMP-1 81
MMT 55
MRSA (Methylcillin Resistant Staph.
        Aureus) 49
multidrug-resistant pumps 48
    MDRs 49
mutations, preventing and reversing 12
myasthenia gravis 35
mylenation of axons 89
myocarditis, viral infection 59
myth 33
    herpes viruses 33
    varicella (chicken pox/shingles) 33

N

N-APP (amyloid precursor protein) 73
National Institutes of Health 89
natural killer cells 78
necrosis 50
nephropathy 23, 25
nerve growth-promoting factor 74
nerve injuries 86
neurite growth 89
neurites, regeneration of after brain
        injuries 67
neurons 66, 67, 71
NF-kappaB 31, 54, 55, 61, 64, 81
non-insulin dependent diabetes
        mellitus (NIDDM).
        See diabetes, Type 2
nutritional metabolic inefficiencies 22
    ability to create Vitamin A 22

O

organically raised food 45
organochloride pesticides
    breast cancer 42

organochlorides 42
organ transplant surgery 12
osteoarthritis 91
osteoblasts 87
osteoporosis 15, 40, 87
   fracture healing 40
oxidation 27

P

Panax notoginseng (tian qi) 40
   addition of 31
   EPO generation 40
   marrow stem cell production 40
pancreatic beta cells 19
Parkinson's Disease (PD) 69, 71
pericytes 30
peripheral nerves 74
   injured 74
peripheral neuropathy 23, 30, 74
pesticides 42
   carcinogenic 43
   organochloride 43
   organophosphates 43
   organophosphate toxicity, reducing 43
   synthetic and children 46
pneumonia 33
polonium 44
Polygonum multiflorum/Reynoutria
     multiflora. *See* he shou wu
polysaccharides 9
   amount of 9
polyunsaturated oils 22
   cooking 22
poor wound healing 23
prednisone 35, 91
pregnancy 34
premature aging 23
progenitor cells 80
prostaglandin 22
protein p53 (cellular tumor antigen) 49
psoriasis 93

Q

Qi 7
quality of life, increase 52

R

radiation 15, 47
   necrosis 50
radiation therapy 35, 47
radon 45
reactive oxygen species (ROS) 82
red blood cell count, increase 35
rehmanniae 30
reperfusion injury 60, 67
retinopathy 23, 31
retinopathy, diabetic 31
rheumatoid arthritis 91
rhinitis 92

S

safety of astragalus 11
sage (Salvia miltiorrhiza) 64
salmon
   Atlantic farmed 42
   wild 42
saponin content 9
saponins 9
scarring, reduced 86
selenium 13
Shannong Bencao 14
Shennong Bencao Jing 7
Shen Qi Da Bu Wan 96
Shen Qi Wu Wei Zi Wan 96
singlet oxygen 32
skin inflammatory diseases, reducing 92
Society of Integrative Oncology 58
soft tissue injuries 14, 86
sorbitol 31
sperm, motility of 85
statin drugs 62
stellate cells 75
stem cells 80
stress syndromes 15
strokes 14, 66

cerebral vascular accidents 66
substantia nigra 70
sugar per year 19
sunburn induced skin cancer 81
super oxide 32
superoxide dismutase (SOD) 69
swainsonines 13
systemic lupus 15

T

TA-65 10
TA65 83, 84
Tau proteins 73
Telomeres 83
The Web That Has No Weaver 8
thymocytes 37
thymus gland 37
Tian Qi 31
TIMP-1 81, 88
tinnitus 87
   ear ringing 88
tissue rejection 33
   astragalus prevented 33
Toll-Like Receptor 4 (TLR4) 61
toxoplasmosis 34
transforming growth factors 24
transplanted tissue 33
Treg cells (T regulator cells) 55
triglycerides 64
triple negative tumors 56
tuberculosis 35
Tumor Necrosis Factor 34
tumor necrosis factor-alpha 90
tumor necrosis factor alpha, NF-
      kappaB 31
tumor necrosis factors 24

U

Ultraviolet A (UVA) 81
ultraviolet B (UVB) 81

V

vincristine 48
viruses 17, 60
   adenovirus 60
   coxsackie 60
Vytorin 64

W

white blood cell count, increase 35

X

xanthines 69

Y

Yu Ping Feng Wan 97

Z

zinc 69

ABOUT THE AUTHOR

After graduating from San Diego State University with a degree in Natural Resource Management, Kimball Chatfield began his formal training in herbal medicine in Naturopathic medical college. He then attended the California Acupuncture College. He received his doctorate in traditional Chinese medicine researching the healing effects of acupuncture in pesticide poisoning. He has taught acupuncture, herbal medicine, and clinical nutrition at three acupuncture colleges and most recently taught Botanical Medicine and Medicinal Plants of the Sierra Nevada at Lake Tahoe Community College. He has authored numerous scientific technical articles, reports, and journal papers, as well as the book *Medicine From the Mountains: Medicinal Plants of the Sierra Nevada.* He maintains a busy natural health care practice in South Lake Tahoe. He lives in the Sierra Nevada county of Alpine in California.

Dr. Chatfield is available for e-mail consultation on the use of astragalus in clinical settings: tahoeacupuncture@gmail.com

Made in the USA
San Bernardino, CA
01 August 2014